Understanding and Effectively Utilizing Experiential Therapy

Understanding and Effectively Utilizing Experiential Therapy

A Mindfulness and Trauma Sensitive Approach to Extending Talk Therapy

Julie Anne Laser
and
Nicole Nicotera

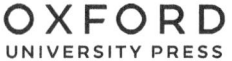

OXFORD
UNIVERSITY PRESS

OXFORD
UNIVERSITY PRESS

Oxford University Press is a department of the University of Oxford.
It furthers the University's objective of excellence in research, scholarship,
and education by publishing worldwide. Oxford is a registered trade mark of
Oxford University Press in the UK and in certain other countries.

Published in the United States of America by Oxford University Press
198 Madison Avenue, New York, NY 10016, United States of America.

CIP data is on file at the Library of Congress

ISBN 9780197757550

DOI: 10.1093/9780197757581.001.0001

Printed by Integrated Books International, United States of America

The manufacturer's authorised representative in the EU for product safety is
Oxford University Press España S.A. of el Parque Empresarial San Fernando
de Henares, Avenida de Castilla, 2 - 28830 Madrid (www.oup.es/en)

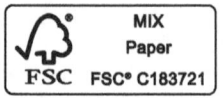

MIX
Paper
FSC FSC® C183721

Contents

Contents

Chapter 1
Introduction

Psychotherapy has been studied now for almost a century, and its effectiveness in treating mental health issues has been validated (Hill & Norcross, 2023). In essence, psychotherapy helps individuals understand, balance, and grow in the aftermath of unwanted or unhealthy experiences. Clinical therapy or psychotherapy has been associated with a host of benefits for many people. It has been found to be more effective than prescribing anti-depressants for anxiety or depression (Cronin et al., 2020; Watson, 2022). Psychotherapy has been linked to the interruption of suicidal thoughts (Freedenthal, 2021) and movement past the crisis. Clinical therapy has been found to ease the symptoms of trauma and to aid in recovery from memories and experiences that have haunted individuals (Herman, 1992, 2015). Psychotherapy changes people's lives for the better.

The effectiveness of psychotherapy comes from the biological and developmental understanding that humans at their core are relational, and from birth forward they need both nurture and education to function at their best (Duncan et al., 2010). Psychotherapy provides a nurturing relationship where the client is heard, seen, understood, and validated in their thoughts, feelings, and behavior. Additionally, clinical therapy educates the client about new strategies, new ways of reframing and thinking, methods to evaluate unhelpful thoughts, feelings, and behavior, and important science-based information about human development, mental health and mental illness, addictions, relationships, and different modalities to effect change. Thus, clinical therapy provides both the nurturing relationship and the education to support the growth that humans need to effect positive change in their own lives.

To be most effective in clinical therapy, clients need to be met where they are emotionally, culturally, and physically by the therapist. Therefore, different therapy modalities work better for different people. This book is primarily about the clinical modality of Experiential Therapy with the addition of mindfulness practices and a trauma-sensitive lens. We have defined Experiential Therapy as "a guided activity, a game, a mental puzzle to work out, time in nature, or a physical challenge to support clinical growth" (Laser & Nicotera, 2021, p. 194). Experiential Therapy provides hands-on, engaged,

Understanding and Effectively Utilizing Experiential Therapy. Julie Anne Laser and Nicole Nicotera, Oxford University Press. © Oxford University Press (2025). DOI: 10.1093/9780197757581.003.0001

holistic experiences aimed at exploring, better understanding, and resolving clinical issues. The *experience* is a conduit that gives rise to words, thoughts, feelings, and future actions that the client would not have found through traditional talk therapy alone.

What Is Experiential Therapy?

As stated already, Experiential Therapy is a guided activity, a game, a mental puzzle to work out, time in nature, or a physical challenge that is used in a clinical framework. Often the Experiential Therapy activity will support the client to "let down their guard" and be fully present in the Experiential Therapy activity, which is why it pairs so well with mindfulness practices, which we will discuss later in the chapter. The clients are not over-thinking themselves, or over-thinking the situation; they are fully present in the Experiential Therapy activity and thus they are who they really are—not a version of themselves because they are in a clinical situation. This allows the clients to engage more fully in the process of therapy and to do so authentically. Often how the client is behaving, thinking, acting, and/or feeling in the Experiential Therapy activity gives rise to insights about current or past experiences, current or past events, people in (or who were in) their lives, their behaviors, their emotions, their thinking, and their reactions to the behaviors of others. We use the term *clinical segues* to describe the transfer of insights from Experiential Therapy activities to insights into their lives outside of therapy.

Clinical Segues

Clinical segues can create new knowledge and insights about how clients are currently leading their lives and how they want to, need to, or can make changes in their lives. Clinical segues transfer the learning from what just happened in the Experiential Therapy activity to what can be taken with them today, tomorrow, and always. Sometimes these clinical segues allow for epiphanies to occur. Clinical segues can focus on new insights into who a person really is, which may include: What is important to them? What can they control in their lives? What strengths do they actually possess? Who in their lives can they count on? What do they really want to do in their lives? What makes them happy? What are the next steps to make their goals a reality? Who really knows them? Who really understands them? Whom can they ask for help? Who will support them in times of need? What have they been hiding from themselves? What have they been hiding from others and why?

What have they been holding on to that they don't need any longer? What are they grieving? Why do they feel shame? Why do they feel loss? Why do they feel abandonment? What makes them anxious? What makes them feel lonely? What makes them feel frustrated? Thus, a myriad of clinical issues can be asked, considered, answered, and fully discussed using Experiential Therapy.

While traditional talk therapy can also support the exploration of new insights, related to the questions listed above, in Experiential Therapy the client uncovers insights from an active, kinesthetic experience followed by a clinical segue, instead of the immediacy of cognitive processing and verbalizing required by talk therapy. Thus, a myriad of clinical issues can be questioned, considered, answered, and fully discussed using Experiential Therapy in way that can be exceptionally helpful for clients who experience the world more kinesthetically or who may have cognitive-emotional defenses that hamper the efforts of insight-oriented talk therapy. For example, when working with a family that is experiencing a disagreement, the Experiential Therapist may use an Experiential Therapy activity called the *human knot*.[1] The family members stand in a circle, place one hand toward the center and grasp someone else's hand and then each one places their other hand in the circle and grasps a different family member's hand so that their arms are intertwined and linked in a knot. The family works together to *untie* the knot without letting go of each other's hands. The Experiential Therapy clinician assists the family in processing both during the activity and afterward through *clinical segues* to uncover, for instance: What had to happen for them to undo the knot? What made the knot get more tangled? How difficult was it for them to not lose each other's hands? What would it mean to let go of each other's hands? Did they act like a team? Did they cooperate? Did members try to sabotage each other during the process? Did they trust each other during the process? Did all members contribute? Did all members speak? Were all members heard? Did all members feel that their contributions were valued? What did they have to do to be successful? Did they agree with what they needed to do to be successful? What were they thinking and feeling during and after the activity? Which actions, thoughts, and feelings can be applied to untying the *knots* of their family disagreements? How can they practice that in the subsequent clinical sessions and in their life outside of therapy?

Additionally, the human knot experience gives the family a metaphor they can apply when they experience the next *knot* in their family functioning outside of therapy. How do they proceed? How do they untie the *knot*?

---

[1] The idea of the human knot and other activities named in this book are commonly used across many fields for different purposes, but to our knowledge, their origins are not attributed to any individual.

How do they reduce the likelihood that *knots* will occur in the family, or when they do occur, how can they best be untied? How do they move to greater harmony in the family? The *human knot* is just one example of how Experiential Therapy offers an exploration, clinical segues, and metaphors for the clients' concerns. These clinical segues and metaphors can be revisited during therapy and used as a common language for the family at home.

By being physically, emotionally, and mentally engaged in the activity, the clients can more fully process the experience. They are using their complete selves. This full involvement in the activity allows for clients to make greater gains in fewer sessions than in talk therapy alone (Laser, 2022). Thus, Experiential Therapy promotes greater well-being by engaging clients' physical, emotional, and cognitive selves together holistically.

How Is Experiential Therapy Different From Traditional Talk Therapy?

Experiential Therapy is an alternative to traditional talk therapy because the clients and clinicians are actively and physically engaged in activities that foster introspection, change, well-being, and resilience. Movement and/or being outdoors creates an atmosphere where clinical conversations are often more natural and less forced than in an office or online. Due to this, clients are often more open and willing to do the work of clinical therapy. The clients frequently allow themselves to be more vulnerable and more authentic in Experiential Therapy clinical sessions rather than in the confines of an office or on a computer platform, where they "believe" there are prescribed behaviors and roles of the client and clinician. It allows both the client and clinician to be more of their genuine selves. The client does not feel so observed, evaluated, and analyzed, and the therapist can remove themselves from being the "all-knowing sage" in the room (which hopefully, they are not doing, but the client may be interpreting them that way). In Experiential Therapy, the clinician truly becomes the guide for the client.

In Experiential Therapy, the client is freed from searching for words to explain their specific problems or issues; instead, they actively present their problems and issues through involvement in the Experiential Therapy activities. This allows the clinician to better ascertain exactly what happens for the client, instead of interpreting what the client is saying. This is particularly salient if the client cannot find the exact words to describe the situation or has a social desirability bias to portray themselves in a particular light. Thus, the Experiential Therapy activities act as a catalyst for both the therapist and the client to gain insights into the client's actions, thoughts, frustrations, sensitivities, and feelings.

Experiential Therapy offers an exploration of clinical segues and metaphors of the clients' concerns, allowing them to safely move out of their comfort zone and into a place of new insights of self-discovery, confidence building, self-awareness, and new methods of how to cope with issues in their lives. These metaphors, such as the *human knot*, can be used in and out of therapy to provide a common language not only for the clients and therapist during a therapy session, but also for the clients to use outside of sessions to become aware, to acknowledge, and to intervene when the issues/problems/negative thoughts or feelings are encroaching upon their daily lives. The use of the metaphors also helps the clients gain insight into the distance they have made in their own journey to greater mental health, resilience, and well-being. The metaphors can act as a baseline for where they were when they initiated Experiential Therapy and where they are in the present.

Experiential Therapy also allows the clinician to get real-time feedback on how these issues manifest in different scenarios depending on the Experiential Therapy activity. This creates opportunities for the clinician and clients to collaborate on assessment and reassessment and to make changes and fine-tune how to best support the clients' goals through Experiential Therapy. This can often happen in real time during the session as part of the clinical process.

Challenge by Choice

In Experiential Therapy, we use a "challenge by choice" philosophy (Rohnke, 1977, 1984) to determine the client's level of participation. As a guide in the process of psychotherapy, we follow the client's lead as to the pace and level of involvement in the Experiential Therapy activities. Through challenge by choice, the client is always empowered to make a choice about whether they participate, their duration of participation, and the quality of their participation. The clinician *always* follows the lead of the client. The client can choose to fully participate, less than fully participate, or even just watch the activity from the sidelines. The client is never coerced or enticed to join in the activity. Most of the time, the client will enjoy participating, but if the client is reticent, the time that they need to feel comfortable is time well spent. It does not matter for Experiential Therapy if the client climbed the mountain with the Experiential Therapist or just sat on the bench at the trailhead. In either instance, it is always challenge by choice, and whichever choice the client makes can be fashioned into clinical segues that increase learning and growth.

If the client chooses not to participate fully, that is a clinical segue and a point to discuss. For instance, how in other spheres of their life do they participate or not? How do they feel about that level of participation? What do they believe they gain and lose by their level of participation? This helps to make challenge by choice an opportunity to learn about the client and to assess how over time they increase their level of participation.

We explain challenge by choice and how therapy takes place in Experiential Therapy with clients through a discussion of *comfort zones*. This is similar to Briere's therapeutic window (Briere, 2002). Briere explains, "this window refers to that psychological location between overwhelming exposure and excessive avoidance wherein therapeutic interventions are most helpful" (Briere, 2002, p. 10). Interventions that are below the therapeutic window, such as avoiding discussion or deflecting, are what we call being in the *relax zone* where little growth and insights can happen. The relax zone may be a lovely respite for the client, but generally it is not a location that is worthwhile for clinical intervention. Conversely, interventions that provide too much intensity or could activate traumatic responses or triggers put the client in what we call the *panic zone*. Entering the panic zone can have a very negative impact on the client and their progress. In the panic zone, if therapy is too intense, the client may feel they need to avoid or discontinue therapy for their own self-preservation. Thus, optimally, to make strides in Experiential Therapy the movement or pace of therapy is to keep the client in the *learning zone*, or within the therapeutic window (Briere, 2002), where insights and growth can happen. Throughout the Experiential Therapy sessions, the clinician should assess the client's *physical arousal* (breathing rate, reddening of the face, tightening of the muscles of the face and hands, perspiration, anxious movement, gesturing) and *verbal arousal* (coherence in communication, speed of communication, swearing, ability to speak or shutting down from speaking) to support the client's staying in the *learning zone.*

In Experiential Therapy, we ask clients to let us know if they are in the relax zone, learning zone, or panic zone. This helps to get a quick read from the clients during activities, more than just attending to their verbal and physical arousal. Importantly, it serves as a moment for the client to self-evaluate and connect to themselves. This in itself is extremely essential for clients who have experienced trauma, who may not normally connect to their inner selves because it has caused pain in the past. This helps clients begin to understand that checking in with their body does not have to invoke pain and can be beneficial and self-protective, which we will further discuss. These terms also help the client understand how their inner feelings are always irrevocably linked to the activities in their lives. Additionally, as we move through subsequent Experiential Therapy sessions, we have a shared language to ascertain how they are doing in Experiential Therapy, as well as to help them see the progress they have made in being able to spend more time in the learning zone as sessions progress.

Challenge by Choice and Trauma Histories

Trauma can result from life-threatening experiences such as living in a war zone, being trafficked, watching interpersonal violence occur between parents, being in a car accident, being a victim of physical or emotional abuse, losing a loved one, being in a natural disaster, being a target of a crime or assault, as well as from socially-emotionally threatening experiences such as witnessing a murder or cruelty to others, or being targeted or bullied for minoritized identities. Trauma lives in the body (Van Der Kolk, 2014). Through movement and body awareness, the brain can be reprogramed to how it interprets and understands the traumatic event (Van Der Kolk, 2014). Thus, activities that promote movement and body awareness, such as Experiential Therapy, enlist the whole person and can support post-traumatic growth, as long as they are done in a trauma-sensitive manner and the person is ready to engage in the activity.

Experiential Therapy supports a trauma-sensitive approach in clinical therapy because the challenge by choice philosophy means that the client is always in control of their destiny. This is extremely important for clients who have experienced trauma. Choice is not an element of traumatic experiences, and some clients will need to reclaim making choice or even claim making choice for the first time. When an individual understands and is able to have a sense of agency over choice, then challenge by choice gives them the total control to participate, their duration of participation, and the quality of their participation. Through Experiential Therapy, they begin to experience a sense of control of their lives during the therapy session instead of merely acting or reacting to other's behaviors or requests. This, in itself, is a huge step forward in their own recovery.

Sometimes, due to current or past trauma, a client's inner feelings and external experiences have become disconnected, and they may present with somatic reactions or dissociative experiences. Thus, the discussion of comfort zone may prove to be a particularly important topic in their recovery. Due to this disconnection between their inner feelings and outer activities, they may need time to be able to process and articulate whether they are in the relax, learning, or panic zone and may need help in being able to ascertain what each zone feels like in their body and mind.

We use an Experiential Therapy activity that helps clients experience and assess their comfort zones, which are often discussed in future sessions as well. We ask the group to make a large circle and to stand about six feet apart from each other. We then ask them to take two giant steps in and ask what they experience; we continue with two more giant steps in and ask what they experience, until they are practically touching shoulders. We also give the choice for clients to stop taking steps if they experience discomfort at any point. In this activity the clinician facilitates a clinical segue to assist clients in recognizing that each person may have a different experience of what they deem as comfortable contact, close contact, and the panic zone. For example, some clients may experience the panic zone when they are six feet apart, some may experience it when they are touching shoulders, and others may not experience it at all. The experiential awareness here is for each individual to notice what they deem as their comfort and panic zones and to honor their needs to be sufficiently distant from others so they can feel comfortable. We bring this experience back to the concept of challenge by choice so that clients with or without a trauma background gain or regain agency and autonomy or choice in their life, first in the clinical sessions, and then to be able to replicate and generalize this in other spheres of their lives.

Challenges of Challenge by Choice

It should be stated that by embracing the challenge by choice philosophy, there are some challenges. The first challenge is that clients may not challenge themselves at all. Does this happen? Yes, but seldomly. Usually when it does, clients may have a trauma history that is unknown to the clinician and may require more time to observe how the Experiential Therapy activity goes, with an option to engage more when they are ready. Other clients may just need a moment to ask questions and gain a better understanding of what is expected of them to participate in the Experiential Therapy activity, with the reassurance that they can choose to opt out of the activity if they assess they are moving into the panic zone. If any client experiences a lot of stress, there are two possible solutions: either discontinue the activity, or have them to observe the activity to see if they might decide to participate. If a client is apprehensive, it can help to have them set a marker for how they will know if they need to discontinue the activity, so they are empowered to make the choice that fits for them. In addition, the clinician is using their honed skills of observation and knowledge of how stress can appear for people and checking in with apprehensive clients who appear to be on the edge of stress.

Conversely, some clients may receive too much positive peer pressure to join in the Experiential Therapy activity when internally they are not ready to do so. This can happen when the client has been cajoled by overly enthusiastic peers or family members to join in the Experiential Therapy activity when they really just want to sit on the sidelines. In this scenario, it is incumbent upon the Experiential Therapist to reiterate the challenge by choice philosophy and to remind all participants that everyone is equipped with their own ability to decide how they choose to participate.

Another issue that may occur is that since clients can set their endpoint, they may give up prematurely and later regret it. In these circumstances, if time allows, we would begin the Experiential Therapy activity anew and have them participate until its conclusion. This gives the client a great sense of accomplishment and persevering through the task. Sense of accomplishment and perseverance can also be used as themes for the clinical segues, as to when and how they have been successful in the past at completing tasks or persevering, or conversely when and how they have not been successful in the past. Additionally, clinical segues on past regrets of not completing tasks or not taking opportunities that they were afforded can be fruitful clinical segues and give many insights into where they understand they are currently and how they got there.

Some clients may set goals for participation in the Experiential Therapy activity too high for them and may not reach their goal or may be unable to finish the activity. This calls for an important clinical segue so the client can explore the experience of not reaching a goal or completing something. In the next session, you could begin the Experiential Therapy activity where the client left off, or set aside time to do the activity again. In either instance, clinical segues that could ensue are conversations around closure, finishing activities, foreclosure of activities or plans that have not been completed in their lives, time management, and perhaps perfectionism.

Other clients may rush to completion of the Experiential Therapy activity and thus may become frustrated with the activity or with each other. In impatient groups or for particular group members who are impatient, the desire to complete the task may be stronger than experiencing the process of doing the activity. As the Experiential Therapy clinician, it is our job to ascertain how much frustration is taking place in the group and whether this is impeding the group members from remaining in the learning zone or moving into the panic zone. It should be said that some frustration may be good to evaluate how group members cope with stress and frustration outside of therapy. However, if they are coming close to the precipice of the panic zone, then we can remind the group that each group member always operates with challenge by choice and that any choice they make is acceptable. If it is just one pushy or frustrated member of the group or family, often the group will self-correct the group member, so that they are more in line with the other group members. These can be very interesting clinical segues to discuss after the activity and to explore how each client deals with stress, frustration, and overbearing behavior outside of therapy and what strategies they use, how the strategies work for them, and in what venues they work better. It is also quite an informative assessment tool with families to ascertain who are the task and emotional leaders of the family and how the family works under pressure.

Why May a Clinician Want to Use Experiential Therapy?

There are many clients that can benefit from the modality of Experiential Therapy. Some of the client characteristics that are particularly efficacious for the use of Experiential Therapy are: clients who have difficulty telling their trauma story; clients who are anxious or worried about being judged or evaluated; clients who believe clinical therapy is unnatural or strange; clients who feel uneasy about needing to fill the therapy session with talk; clients who have trouble sitting for 50+ minutes (which includes ADHD clients); clients who have trouble focusing; clients who have trouble making or keeping eye contact; clients who feel uncomfortable in a small office or online; and clients who feel stifled when not moving their hands, feet, or bodies.

When the client moves into a more natural environment, the energy that was being used to maintain themselves in the more sterile clinical office or online environment is lessened, and that energy can then be used to gain greater insights into their thinking, behavior, emotions, reasoning, and rationale. Thus, by providing clients with a more natural and less artificial or sterile environment, where clients feel more comfortable, less stressed, less awkward, less defensive, less observed or viewed, less assessed or evaluated, less shamed or feeling guilty, or less judged, they can make greater strides to healthier functioning. For these clients, we have found that Experiential Therapy is a very effective modality.

How Does It Fit Comfortably With Mindfulness-Based Approaches?

Mindfulness-based approaches originate from Buddhism, Ayurveda, and Traditional Chinese Medicine (Lee et al., 2009). These have been brought to the Western world in various ways, most notably by the Dalai Lama's efforts to connect with practitioners and scholars at Emory University (https://tibet.emory.edu/) and Richard Davidson, PhD, at the Center for Healthy Minds at the University of Wisconsin, Madison (https://www.centerhealthyminds.org/). Mindfulness approaches take the stance that "problems are viewed as opportunities for growth" and encourages clients to understand problems as part of life, that life will always bring challenges, and that the goal is to learn how to navigate them (Lee et al., 2009, p. 312). This stance pairs well with Experiential Therapy, which has the goal of learning through experience and applying that learning to the next challenges one will face.

Pairing Experiential Therapy with mindfulness practices further increases the depth and breadth of the experience. Mindfulness brings clients into present-moment awareness of the Experiential Therapy activity itself, so they are totally engaged in the present moment of the activity and the feelings, thoughts, and body sensations that arise during it. Mindfulness practices have been validated for supporting healing, recovery from trauma, well-being, and resilience. For example, the capacity for mindfulness is associated with quality of life (Thieleman & Cacciatore, 2014; Thomas, 2012; Thomas & Otis, 2010; Thompson et al., 2014), perceived stress (Feng et al., 2019), emotion regulation (Kral et al., 2018), and positive academic functioning (Beauchemin et al., 2008; Howell & Buro, 2011; Shao & Skarlicki, 2009). In addition, evidence supports a connection between mind-body activities and coping with stress and skills for self-regulation (Leitch, 2017).

Mindfulness interventions help people to regulate the automatic fight, flight, freeze responses of the nervous system (Marchand, 2014) and to build the capacity to regulate the challenges of trauma histories (Leitch, 2017). In other words, pairing mindfulness practices with Experiential Therapy fosters clients' ability to recognize when they are nearing the panic zone and to skillfully manage the experience so they can more successfully engage with the therapy process and bring themselves into the learning zone or relax zone, depending on what they need in that moment.

Our Version of Experiential Therapy

The name Experiential Therapy comes from the experiential learning tradition that was first articulated by John Dewey in 1939. Experiential learning posits that students learn by doing and reflecting on their experiences. Experiential learning honors the student's current and past knowledge and experiences, engages them in an activity where they apply that knowledge to new real-life experiences, and then after the activity, engages the student in reflection to synthesize the new learning and to create new knowledge. Experiential Therapy follows a similar process, but with a focus on the client's clinical challenges so they can gain insights into conceptualizing the problems in their own life, increasing problem-solving strategies, understanding possible flaws in their past thinking about their problems, and increasing self-discovery of their resilience, strength, self-knowledge, and adaptability in new situations.

Some of the Experiential Therapy activities discussed in this book were created by the authors themselves specifically for Experiential Therapy, but many activities come from a long tradition of outdoor recreation and have been used to create teachable moments with students, campers, and groups in the vein of experiential education. These activities are enhanced in the therapeutic processes of Experiential Therapy.

Experiential Therapy is always done by a mental health clinician whose training equips them with tools, knowledge, and skills pertinent to mental health, social-emotional issues, or other complex presentations such as trauma that are outside the training and realm of experiential educators. This is where experiential learning moves to Experiential Therapy, where clients engage first in an experiential learning activity and then, through clinical segues by the Experiential Therapist, develop insight into how their behavior, thinking, voice, and comfort level replicate or do not replicate their "real-world life and issues." We have found that when a trained mental health clinician combines experiential learning activities with clinical segues, this serves as a catalyst to clinical progress. We understand that not everyone enjoys being active and moving during clinical therapy, but many do, and for those clients and clinicians, Experiential Therapy is an innovative approach to resolving their issues.

Experiential Therapy has not been attributed to one person, like Dialectical Behavior Therapy (DBT) to Marsha Linehan, or Eye Movement Desensitization and Reprocessing (EMDR) to Francine Shapiro. Experiential Therapy is more akin to how Aaron Beck has been labeled the "father" of Cognitive Behavior Therapy (CBT), but later and currently, many clinicians and scholars have practiced and written about CBT in different situations with different populations and have created a plurality of CBT publications, trainings, and techniques. That is, Experiential Therapy is more like CBT, where several people have written about it and have their versions of it. We know that there are other practices labeled Experiential Therapy, such as drama therapy or psychodrama. In fact, the American Addiction Centers catalog Experiential Therapy under Expressive Therapies (https://americanaddictioncenters.org/therapy-treatment/experiential), which include drama therapy/psychodrama, music therapy, art therapy, play therapy, poetry therapy, animal-assisted therapies, and adventure therapies.

Our use of the term Experiential Therapy arises out of adventure therapies but takes a clinical, trauma-sensitive approach, requires mental-health-trained clinicians, and does not require hiking, camping, or otherwise spending time in the wilderness or even outdoors, where many people who have experienced trauma become activated. We understand that we are not the only voices out there that use the term Experiential Therapy, but we have created our unique version of it. We do believe that—just as CBT is a plurality of writing, techniques, and trainings about, at its essence, *how our thoughts get in the way of our behavior*—Experiential Therapy at its essence involves *using the whole person during clinical therapy*, though how this is done differs between practitioners and scholars, creating a plurality of writing, training, and techniques. This book is our version of Experiential Therapy, drawn from the robust experiential learning tradition.

Experiential Therapy Activity

To further illustrate Experiential Therapy, throughout the book we will be sharing specific Experiential Therapy activities, that can be easily replicated by the reader. You will notice with every activity we use a 10-step outline for Experiential Therapy: name of activity; time duration; purpose/objective; age/gender/cultural considerations; equipment/materials needed; risk assessment; framing questions; directions for activity; clinical segues and questions; for whom would this activity be appropriate, and for whom would it not be appropriate? We will go into greater detail regarding the characteristics of the 10 steps in Chapter 7, "Structuring Experiential Therapy Interventions." The first activity is called "Sunshine in a Can." It is an activity that would be appropriate for a newly formed Experiential Therapy group. As the book continues we will share activities that support group development, increased group cohesion, and opportunities to support more vulnerable sharing in group activities.

Sunshine in a Can

Time Duration: 20–40 minutes

Purpose/Objective: Problem-solving and communication activity

Age/Gender/Cultural Considerations: 10 years and up, minimum of four participants, no gender or cultural considerations

Equipment/Materials Needed: Coffee can, inner bike tube or resistance band, one 10-foot length of rope per participant, jug, funnel, container of water

Tie the bike tube/resistance band into a loop that tightly fits near the top of the coffee can.

Tie one end of each 10-foot rope to the bike tube/resistance band that is around the coffee can to make a coffee can transporting device.

Thus, if there are five participants, there are five lengths of rope coming from the bike tube/resistance band which is tied around the coffee can.

Risk Assessment: Minimal risk: to prevent rope burn, participants may not wrap rope around their hands. Participants' feet must stay on the ground.

Framing: (This is how you explain the activity to participants)

The can is filled with sunshine (filled with water).

Your team must safely transport the sunshine in the can to be saved for a rainy day.

You must then safely pour the sunshine into the jug.

You will need to fully fill the jug where the sunshine will be stored.

Directions for Activity: (Explain the rules of the activity to the participants)

1. Transport the contents of the coffee can to the jug and funnel that are placed at some distance from the coffee can.
2. Must use the coffee can and ropes to transport the contents.
3. Must hold the ropes at their end (keeping a 10-foot radius away from the can)
4. Must pour water from coffee can into the jug.
5. Participants are not allowed to use their hands or selves to pour the water from the coffee can to the jug. The funnel in the jug will make pouring the water somewhat easier.
6. The activity is completed when the jug is filled with water.
7. This may take several times of moving the coffee can by the ropes to the jug, and pouring the water into the jug, returning to the starting point of the coffee can and having it refilled with water, until the jug is fully filled with water.

Clinical Segues: What skills did the group need to have in order to transport the sunshine? If you pulled too hard on the ropes, what happened? What happened if group members did not work together? How does this apply in real life? Did everyone offer suggestions of how they could move the can to the jug? Did everyone offer suggestions of how they could pour the water into the jug? Were suggestions listened to by all? How is this like other venues in your life? Was there a leader of the group? Were you the leader? Raise your hand if you thought of the solution before the leader did, but did not speak up? What kept you from speaking up? Do you speak up when you have suggestions? Why or why not? Did your leader solicit ideas or just use their ideas? Did the leader of the group change through the activity? What made your group successful? What made your group less successful? What did you learn about your communication style? What did you learn about the communication style of other group members? Did you become frustrated and why? Did others become frustrated and why? How did you work as a team? How did you feel about your group members?

For Whom Would This Activity Be Appropriate, and for Whom Would It Not Be Appropriate?

Sunshine in a Can is an Experiential Therapy activity that works well with families and groups. It generally can be used as an earlier activity in the process of Experiential Therapy. There are two major issues that the group needs to figure out when they are doing the activity: (1) how to walk with the can, and (2) how to pour the water into the jug. The first issue, walking with the can, the group members need to come to understand that they have to hold onto their rope with enough tension to pick up the can filled with water, but not too much tension or the can will slip through the bike tube/resistance band, and they will need to return to the beginning of the course to get the can refilled with sunshine (water). Additionally, if a single group member pulls too heavily on the rope to try to control the direction or with not enough strength, the can will also fall through. Therefore, all members need to walk with the can to move forward. Thus, this is a great opportunity for clinical segues to discuss communication, cooperation, acting as a team, and frustration tolerance.

Second, once they reach the jug, they need to come to the understanding that they are going to need to move carefully together to raise one side of the can to be able to pour the water into the jug. They can do this by assigning some members to walk around other members to shorten some of the ropes so that they can pour the water. If they do not do this and they pull too hard, the can will fall through or they will not be able to have enough precision to get the water into the jug. This usually takes some time and experimentation to figure out the strategy. Once again, this is a great opportunity for clinical segues not only about communication, cooperation, acting as a team, and frustration tolerance, but also about brainstorming, trying new ideas, thinking outside of the box, being inventive, promoting one's own ideas, being listened to and being heard, contributing to the team, and completing tasks as a team. Clients who have a hard time being part of a team or have a low frustration tolerance will have a more difficult time with the activity.

Looking Ahead to the Next Chapters

In Chapter 2, we will focus on the foundations of Experiential Therapy in experiential learning. Additionally, we will discuss the theoretical support and research evidence behind the use of Experiential Therapy. Also in Chapter 2, the scientific benefits of being in nature will be discussed, as well as using nature as a clinical partner in wellness. Research on the positive influences of being in nature on health and wellness will be discussed. Finally, we will discuss the differences between Experiential Therapy and wilderness therapy.

In Chapter 3 we will discuss trauma and trauma sensitivity. This will include defining both concepts. The chapter will also highlight how trauma lives in the body and how through activity it can be ameliorated. Skills for educating clients about the window of tolerance and how to put on the brakes between learning zone and panic zone will be further discussed.

Chapter 4, "Integrating Mindfulness with Experiential Therapy," will discuss mindfulness practices. This chapter will share how mindfulness honors traditions, cultures, and systems of medicine from which it arises. Additionally, evidence will be presented of how mindfulness practices support healing and recovery. Benefits of integrating mindfulness practices into Experiential Therapy will be explored, specifically how mindfulness practices and Experiential Therapy are a good fit for working with survivors of trauma.

In Chapter 5, "Fine-Tuning for the Clinician: Capacities for Well-Being and Working Across Identities," we will discuss how we can fine-tune ourselves to practice habits of wellness and to work across the multiple identities of our clients.

In Chapter 6, "Risk Management," we will discuss the risks associated with Experiential Therapy. We will explain how we introduce the idea of Experiential Therapy to our clients and the collaborative exploration of whether it's a good fit. Additionally, risks, both physical and emotional, will be discussed for both the clinician and the client. The difference between foreseeable risks versus unforeseeable risks, including triggers/activation, will be elucidated. We will share with readers the risk-management tools and the checklist we have created and use regularly to ensure that risks are minimized. The importance of careful preparation will be emphasized.

Chapter 7, "Structuring Experiential Therapy Interventions," will discuss the details of how to organize Experiential Therapy activities. A 10-step outline for Experiential Therapy will be presented to support one's thinking and planning for the Experiential Therapy activity. Scaling activities to increase insights over time for clients, decrease effects of trauma, and increase resilience will be shared. Three Experiential Therapy activities will be shared.

In Chapter 8, we will discuss "Experiential Therapy in the Natural Realm." Additional risks and benefits of moving clinical intervention into nature will be shared. We will discuss outdoor interventions by seasons. We share protocols for a wide variety of outdoor activities: walking, hiking, challenge course, road biking, camping, paddleboarding, and snowshoeing.

In Chapter 9, we will discuss "Experiential Therapy in the Virtual Realm." Due to the COVID-19 pandemic, we will discuss how to use virtual technology to do Experiential Therapy. We will discuss how we have had to reconceive Experiential Therapy in a virtual realm. We will share three virtual Experiential Therapy activities in this chapter.

Chapter 10 will discuss Experiential Therapy activities with specific populations: children, youth, couples, and families. We will give multiple examples of Experiential Therapy activities that work with each of these populations.

Chapter 11 will discuss Experiential Therapy with some of the diverse populations we work with: survivors of human trafficking, veterans and military service members, persons with substance use disorders (SUDs), juvenile-justice-involved youth, and grief groups. We will give examples of Experiential Therapy activities that work well with these populations.

Chapter 12 concludes with how to evaluate Experiential therapy's effectiveness in your organization or practice. We will share our Institutional Review Board (IRB)–approved instruments developed for Experiential Therapy research evaluation.

We believe this book will give you the necessary knowledge and skill development to be able to do Experiential Therapy in your own practice and we are excited for you to join us!

Chapter 2
Foundations of Experiential Therapy

Foundations of Experiential Learning in Experiential Therapy

As stated in Chapter 1, experiential learning has been suggested as an integrated way of learning since John Dewey wrote his seminal treatise, *Experience and Education*, in 1939. Experiential learning honors the student's current and past knowledge and experiences, engages them in an activity where they apply that knowledge to new real-life experiences, and then after the activity, engages the student in reflection to synthesize the new learning and to create new knowledge. Dewey states, "what they learn in the way of knowledge and skill in one situation becomes an instrument of understanding and dealing effectively with situations that follow" (Dewey, 1939, p. 42), suggesting that all knowledge builds on itself, and past experiences and thoughts influence current and future thinking. Additionally, new experiences allow for new and novel ways of thinking and new repertoires of how to proceed in unfamiliar situations.

Others applying Dewey's pedagogy of experiential leaning have created a flow chart for supporting experiential learning by going through the steps: (1) experience the activity; (2) share reactions and observations openly; (3) process and analyze the experience; (4) connect the experience to real-life experiences; (5) apply what was learned to similar or different situations (Great Pedagogical Thinkers, 2023).

Dewey also emphasizes that "all human experience is ultimately social: that it involves contact and communication" (Dewey, 1939, p. 32). This suggests that synthesizing new information and ideas is best supported through discussion, with intentional opportunities to mull over the ideas and information with others, to seek alternative ideas, and to engage in an evolving process to form new information and ideas—which sounds remarkably similar to the clinical process; hence the foundational link between experiential learning and clinically oriented Experiential Therapy.

Understanding and Effectively Utilizing Experiential Therapy. Julie Anne Laser and Nicole Nicotera, Oxford University Press. © Oxford University Press (2025). DOI: 10.1093/9780197757581.003.0002

Foundations of Human Ecology in Experiential Therapy

Experiential Therapy helps clients become aware and gain insight into their relationships: within themselves, with others, and the world around them. Thus, Experiential Therapy is philosophically grounded in *ecological theory*, which is the science of interrelationships among living organisms and between organisms in their natural, built, and social environments (Bubolz & Sontag, 1993; Griffore & Phenice, 2001; Hayword, 1994). Ecological theory proposes that the characteristics of an individual in interaction with the characteristics of the environment over time influence the development of that individual as well as the environment (Barrows, 1995; Bubolz & Sontag, 1993; Griffore & Phenice, 2001).

Bronfenbrenner (1979) builds on ecological theory to create the term *human ecology*, which explains the developing person "as a growing dynamic entity that progressively moves into and restructures the milieu in which it resides" (p. 21). The environment transforms and accommodates the individual, and the individual transforms and accommodates the environment. Neither the environment nor the individual is the same due to their interaction (Bronfenbrenner, 1979, 1986, 1989). A human ecological perspective allows the clinician to assess and intervene at multilevel interactions between the client and their environment, whether that environment is within themselves, or between themselves and others in the natural, built, and social environments (Griffore & Phenice, 2001).

Thus, as we develop as human beings, we are continually being transformed by other people and by the natural, built, and social environments, and those other people and environments are also continually being transformed by their interactions with us. This means that we effect change in the environments in which we live/work/go to school/recreate, and those environments influence change in us as well, in a continuous exchange over time. Thus, philosophically, from a *human ecology* lens we are always capable of developing, changing, and growing as well as affecting the world around us. From a trauma-informed perspective, this suggests a lot of hope for moving through and growing past traumatic experiences.

Theoretical Underpinnings of the Benefits of Being in Nature

There is a widely held belief that being in nature does us good. Carl Jung in a lecture in 1928 stated, "Whenever we touch nature we get clean. People who have got dirty through too much civilization take a walk in the woods, or a bath in the sea. They shake off the fetters and allow nature to touch them" (Improvised Life, n.d., para. 1). Many of us are aware that we feel better when we breathe fresh air and experience the beautiful natural world around us. We may feel greater wellness when we are outside. Many have posited that this deep connection to nature has always been with us, and as we have separated ourselves from nature we have made ourselves less healthy and less whole (Buzzell & Chalquist, 2009; Goldsmith, 1998; Hanscom, 2016; Louv, 2008; Mathews, 1991; Merchant, 1999; Plotkin, 2013; Roszak et al., 1995; Selhub & Logan, 2012; Sessions, 1995; Thomashow, 1995; Williams, 2017). Thus, by being in nature, we begin to put the disparate parts of us back together. Williams states, "we think of nature as a luxury not a necessity" (2017, p. 12). In actuality, nature is an important ingredient in our lives for all of us to support holistic well-being and resilience.

Research Findings on the Benefits of Being in Nature

Research has found that active time in nature elevates self-esteem and mood, and the effect was greatest when people were near water (Barton & Pretty, 2010). Interestingly, time in nature did not need to be prolonged (less than an hour) and lower-intensity activities were more beneficial than high-intensity activities (Barton & Pretty, 2010). This has prompted some medical doctors to write prescriptions for more time outside (Jorgensen, 2020). For some individuals this has been very effective (Meredith et al., 2020). For instance, college-age individuals who spent 10 minutes of sitting or walking in natural settings significantly and positively impacted psychological and physiological markers of mental well-being (Meredith et al., 2020).

However, research on "green" prescriptions for children did not find a significant difference between those who received a "green" prescription and those who did not (Christiana et al., 2017). Half of the parents (49%) viewed the "green" prescriptions as beneficial for their children, and those that used the intervention materials at home with their child found it to be even more beneficial (70%) (Christiana et al., 2017). Thus, parents merely telling kids to "go play outside" may have made some parents feel better, but greater change happened when they also were outside with their children.

Other research on forest-bathing further bolsters the healing properties of being in nature. Forest-bathing, which originated in Japan in the 1980s (Furuyashiki et al., 2019) and is now common across numerous countries, "refers to a healing technique that restores the physical and psychological health of the human body through a 'five senses experience' (vision, smell, hearing, touch, and taste) when the body is exposed to a forest environment" (Wen et al., 2019, pp. 1–2). Research demonstrates that forest-bathing can *lower blood pressure* (Ideno et al., 2017), *reduce negative mood* (Tsunetsugu, 2010), *reduce depression and anxiety* (Chun et al., 2017), and *reduce chronic pain and depression* (Han et al., 2016). Forest bathing, with its clear and flexible directions, can easily be incorporated into nature-based Experiential Therapy.

Research Findings of Clinical Experiences in Nature

By being in nature, or just outside the confines of the office, we tap into some of that experience of the benefits of being in nature. But to be in nature and to be working with a trained clinician gives the Experiential Therapy session greater power. Nature-based interventions have been found to reduce *rumination* in clients (Bratman et al., 2015); to be a treatment for *attention-deficit/hyperactivity disorder* (ADHD) (Kuo & Taylor, 2004); to improve *calmness* for clients (Tambyah et al., 2022); to improve *neuro-functioning* (Kettler, 2016; Stillman, 2020); to increase *self-esteem* (Schell et al., 2012); to increase *confidence* (Norton et al., 2023); to improve client *mood* (Tambyah et al., 2022); to increase *creativity* (Atchley et al., 2012; Williams, 2017); to increase feelings of *empowerment* (Tambyah et al., 2022); to improve *immune responses* for clients with illness (Cassella, 2020); to increase *emotional well-being* (Joschko et al., 2023; Rose et al., 2018); to decrease *fear* (Rose et al., 2018); and to increase *self-efficacy and confidence* (Norton et al., 2023; Rose et al., 2018).

Additionally, nature-based clinical interventions increase *peer connectiveness* (Rose et al., 2018; Tambyah et al., 2022); increase *school connectedness* (Rose et al., 2018); and increase *connectedness to nature* (Joschko et al., 2023; Landres et al., 2012). Thus, there are both internal and ecological benefits of therapy outside the confines of the office.

Research on Best Practices for Clinicians to Facilitate Therapy in Nature

Clinicians themselves have found that clients' mood, calmness, feelings of relaxation, a sense of empowerment, and social connections improved when they brought clients outside (Tambyah et al., 2022). However, these same clinicians believed that there were some barriers to nature-based interventions, such as lack of motivation of clients, skepticism of clients, geographic accessibility to nature, as well as organizational barriers such as policies around safety and risk (Tambyah et al., 2022). These are exactly the issues we discuss in Chapters 6, 7, and 8 of this book. Additionally, clients reported the importance of the therapist setting the pace and of a supportive environment (Joschko et al., 2023), which we cover in Chapter 7, as well as setting the pace and supportive environments for clients' diverse needs and with particular populations, which we discuss in Chapters 10 and 11, respectively.

Our Research on the Clinical Benefits of Experiential Therapy

We have also been conducting research and writing about the benefits of Experiential Therapy for clients (Laser, 2022; Laser & Nicotera, 2021; Laser-Maira, 2016; Laser-Maira & Nicotera, 2019; Nicotera & Laser-Maira, 2017). We have found that considered preparation is fundamental for having an effective Experiential Therapy session. The more that we ensure that clients understand the tenets of *challenge by choice* and the concept of *comfort zones* (see Chapter 1), the better the Experiential Therapy session is for them. For instance, in recent research (Laser, 2022), we found that 88% of clients agreed that they left their comfort zone during the Experiential Therapy session and that 88% of clients agreed they were glad that they left their comfort zone. Additionally, leaving their comfort zone had a residual effect; 77% of clients agreed they are more likely to leave their comfort zone in the future (Laser, 2022).

Similar to the other research on nature-based therapy presented, we found many clinical benefits to Experiential Therapy. Seventy-seven percent of clients agreed that their experiences increased their ability to *problem solve* (Laser, 2022). Moreover, 76% of clients agreed that their Experiential Therapy interventions will increase their ability to *make decisions* (Laser, 2022). Most (93%) clients agreed that they *grew as a member* of their Experiential Therapy group (Laser, 2022). *Increased trust* was another benefit of their involvement in Experiential Therapy, with 81% of clients agreeing that their experiences increased their trust in others (Laser, 2022).

Self-discovery also increased for those involved in Experiential Therapy, with 79% of clients agreeing that they learned something new about themselves (Laser, 2022). *Personal growth* was also endorsed by most clients, with

83% of clients agreeing that they grew as an individual (Laser, 2022). *Confidence* also increased for those involved in Experiential Therapy, with 81% of clients agreeing that their experiences increased confidence in themselves (Laser, 2022). Moreover, the clinical gains experienced during therapy were reinforced, with 82% of clients agreeing that they will bring these changes to their personal lives (Laser, 2022). Thus, Experiential Therapy has some robust outcomes for its participants.

Differences Between Experiential Therapy and Wilderness Therapy

There are some philosophical and organizational differences between Experiential Therapy and wilderness therapy. Experiential Therapy is always done by a trained mental health clinician, whereas wilderness therapy is often led by a wilderness guide who may or may not have consultation with a mental health professional. Experiential Therapy always upholds the principles of *challenge by choice*, with the client deciding whether to participate, the level of participation, and the duration of participation. There are never consequences for not participating or not participating fully, or not reaching a certain destination. Experiential Therapy does not require that a person hike, camp, or otherwise spend extended time in the wilderness or even outdoors. The Experiential Therapy activities are not arduous, nor is there ever any suggestion of breaking people down to build them anew, as is often suggested in boot-camp wilderness programs. Experiential Therapy is trauma sensitive and works to help clients move within their comfort zone and learn to make choices that allow them to expand their comfort zone in gradual ways as they are ready, in the context of any current or past trauma.

While scholars in wilderness therapy are considering the importance of trauma sensitivity (e.g., Fisher, 2023; Flom, 2022; Johnson et al., 2020) other recent publications point to deficits in trauma awareness within wilderness therapy programs. For example, Okoren (2022) and Sheets (2022) report that some wilderness therapy programs are known to tell parents and caretakers that extended time in nature will help their troubled teens, but that in reality youth who have been involved in these type of harsh boot camps in the outdoors have found the experience "dehumanizing and taking away their dignity" (Moniuzko, 2022, p. 2). Youth who have been sent to these wilderness therapy programs, often against their consent, frequently have experienced public humiliation, shame, being bullied, physical exhaustion, and have frequent nightmares and post-traumatic stress disorder (PTSD) due to the experience (Okoren, 2022; Sakre, 2021; Sheets, 2022). These wilderness therapy programs offer no initial training for the youth entering the wilderness (Okoren, 2022; Sakre, 2021; Sheets, 2022) and place youth in a wilderness environment with staff who often lack education in mental health therapy and trauma (Sheets, 2022). Frequently, the staff who are in charge of these youth have wilderness skills, but they do not have a foundation of mental health training. Some wilderness therapy programs do have staff consult with mental health clinicians, or the mental health professional comes to do weekly therapy, but that mental health clinician is not commonly embedded as onsite staff at the wilderness therapy facility (Kaplan, 2020). Therefore, when a mental health or other clinical crisis occurs in the wilderness, the youth are often without a trained mental health professional and at a great distance from mental health facilities.

In a large-scale evaluation of wilderness therapy programs, Harper (2017) concluded that there were ethical concerns of wilderness therapy programs that needed further attention. Four years later, in 2021, Harper, Fernee, and Gabrielson completed another review of wilderness therapy programs and found that in most programs, structure and activity details with causal links to outcomes were mostly absent. Thus, there were not any theoretical underpinnings, accepted ongoing practices, generalizable tenets or procedures that were uniformly upheld or completed.

In Conclusion

Experiential Therapy has evolved from the tenets of Dewey and experiential learning, the theoretical underpinnings of human ecology, the theory and research on the benefits of being in nature, and the research on being in nature with a trained clinician. We call what we do Experiential Therapy, as opposed to wilderness therapy, due to wilderness therapy's sometimes punitive, unregulated, non-trauma-informed, and non-therapeutic tendencies. We therefore use the term Experiential Therapy whether we are inside or outside with clients.

Next Chapter

In the next chapter, we will discuss trauma and becoming a trauma-sensitive clinician in Experiential Therapy.

Chapter 3
Trauma and Trauma Sensitivity

What Is Trauma?

Trauma can result from life-threatening experiences such as living in a war zone, surviving a natural or civil disaster, being a victim of human trafficking, or surviving rape or intimate partner violence. Trauma can also result from social-emotional-spirit life-threatening experiences of being targeted due to minoritized identities such as race/ethnicity, gender, sexual orientation, ability, neurodiversity, or faith/religion (Connolly & Sullivan, n.d.). Sue (2010) gives voice to this kind of trauma, labeling it *microaggressive stress*, "defined as race-related, gender-related, or sexual orientation related events or situations that are experienced as a perceived threat to one's biological, cognitive, emotional, psychological, and social well-being, or position in life" (p. 96). Emerson and Hopper (2011) write:

> Human beings are tender creatures. We are born with our hearts open. And some-times our open hearts encounter experiences that shatter us. Sometimes we encounter experiences that so violate our sense of safety, order, predictability, and right, that we feel utterly overwhelmed—unable to integrate, and simply unable to go on as before. Unable to bear reality. We have come to call these shattering experiences trauma. None of us is immune to them. (Emerson & Hopper, 2011, p. xiii)

There is a great likelihood that one or more of your clients will have lived through a recent or past trauma. The experience of trauma is widespread with estimates of around 90% of the U.S. population reporting at least one traumatic event in their life (Kilpatrick et al., 2013). In addition, nearly 75% of the U.S. population reported experiencing one or more adverse childhood events (ACE), which include experiences of violence and may be experienced as traumatic events (Swedo, 2023). There are three categories of ACEs: abuse, neglect, and challenges within one's household (such as intimate partner violence, having a family member in prison, living with a substance-addicted family member) (Centers for Disease Control and Prevention, n.d.). Hence, this chapter focuses specifically on trauma and trauma sensitivity.

Understanding and Effectively Utilizing Experiential Therapy. Julie Anne Laser and Nicole Nicotera,
Oxford University Press. © Oxford University Press (2025). DOI:10.1093/9780197757581.003.0003

Trauma can be fresh in someone's life, having occurred within days or months of when you meet them, or it can be historical, being passed across generations or from the more recent past of childhood. The tricky part is that the person you meet as your client may not be consciously aware of having had traumatic experiences; they may have shut these experiences out as a means of psychological self-protection, which is a common sequela in childhood abuse and traumas. As physician Sister Dang Nghiem (2021) points out, "many people [who survive childhood abuse] literally do not remember the incident or only have vague recollections or snapshots of it; in this case, the nervous system has automatically blocked the experience for self-survival purposes" (p. 225). Regardless of the time frame in which it happened, unprocessed trauma can arise in the body, mind, and spirit, as fresh as when it originally occurred, creating uninvited and unexpected reactions from tears to anger to fear to frustration or rage that might be expressed outwardly and/or experienced internally as depression, anxiety, or in some cases a full-body shutdown, as in entering a freeze state or even fainting (Nghiem, 2021).

Trauma Lives in the Body

The experience of trauma activates the body's natural warning system, the same system that allows us to jump out of the way of an oncoming car without missing a beat. However, after the car passes, we recover, maybe by exhaling a large whoosh of breath and then a slow intake of breath, and the warning system returns to equilibrium or balance (Nghiem, 2021; Van der Kolk, 2014). In trauma, the body's warning system does not return to equilibrium; instead, that early warning system remains activated, and thereafter, unprocessed trauma creates:

> the intense suffering of never truly feeling relaxed, at ease in life, always intensely on guard, with the primitive brain constantly scanning for threat or opportunity. 'Trauma always happens *in the body*. It is a spontaneous mechanism used by the body to stop or thwart further (or future) potential damage . . . An embedded trauma response can manifest as fight, flee, or freeze—or some combination of constriction, pain, fear, dread, anxiety, unpleasant (and/or pleasant thoughts), reactive behaviors, or other sensations and experiences. This trauma then gets stuck in the body—and stays there until it is addressed' (Menakem, 2017, p. 7). When trauma is stuck in the body, our inner sentry is always on watch. (Emerson & Hopper, 2011, p. xv)

Indeed, unprocessed trauma experiences can result in the body's chronic release of stress hormones such as cortisol (Van der Kolk, 2014), almost as if the body were running marathon after marathon without a rest, resulting in chronic outcomes that negatively impact the body, mind, and spirit (Kabat-Zinn, 2013; Van der Kolk, 2014).

Trauma lives in the body and can be triggered as well as ameliorated through physical activity. "In order to change, people [who experience trauma] need to become aware of their sensations and the way their bodies interact with the world around them. Physical self-awareness is the first step to releasing the tyranny of the past" (Van der Kolk, 2014, p. 119). This suggests that Experiential Therapy, which involves varying degrees of physical activity, can trigger unaddressed trauma in clients, but that when done in a trauma-sensitive modality can be healing for trauma survivors as they develop physical awareness and begin to take steps to release the "tyranny of the past" for their bodies. Physical awareness is also called somatic awareness or "'interoception' [which] is a tool that allows us to 'track' the workings of our autonomic nervous system, which is constantly evaluating our inner and outer environment and responding accordingly" (Ozawa-de Silva, 2023, para. 30). The autonomic nervous system is the formal name of the natural early warning system we mentioned at the beginning of this chapter, where fight, fight, freeze, reactions are ignited when danger appears and where the calming reaction occurs when we let out a large, exhaled whoosh of breath, for example after we jump out of the way of a car and realize we are safe (Kabat-Zinn, 2013). Recall that this same early warning system is activated during trauma experiences; however, as we mentioned earlier in this chapter, the system does not return to balance, there is no large, exhaled whoosh of breath and return to equilibrium. When trauma is addressed and survivors develop interoception, they can begin to practice at allowing the sentry that was always on duty to have a rest, to know when danger is imminent and when they are safe in their body, mind, and spirit. Trauma-sensitive movement can be an initial step toward honing the skills for interoception (Emerson & Hopper, 2011).

Trauma-sensitive movement that engages clients in being curious and slowly exploring their physical sensations may foster new body awareness that allows them to reduce the grip of past trauma (Salmon, 2020). Awareness-based movement in a context of curiosity and nonjudgment can help clients increase the capacity to be resilient in the face of unnerving physical and emotional sensation (Emerson & Hopper, 2011). Awareness-based movement and body-mind-spirit practices, such as walking meditation and body scans that do not require clients to verbally share their trauma story, are an important intervention modality because people who have experienced trauma can have great difficulty expressing their experiences in words (Shin et al., 1999). Evidence for this difficulty arises from functional magnetic resonance images (fRMI) of the brain showing that the part of the brain associated with speech and language can shut down during and after trauma (Shin et al., 1999, cited in Stoller et al., 2012, p. 59). The major caveat is that clinicians apply trauma-sensitive concepts and skills in their work with clients as they address their trauma experiences and histories.

Trauma Sensitivity: Concepts

The terms *trauma aware, trauma sensitive*, and *trauma-informed practices/approaches/care* are often used interchangeably (Bartlett, 2021; McConnico et al., 2016), but they are described differently depending on the organization, practitioner, or researcher. For example, the Substance Abuse and Mental Health Services Administration (SAMHSA) uses the term *trauma-informed approach* and defines it from a more global perspective as "inclusive of trauma-specific interventions, whether assessment, treatment or recovery supports, [that] also incorporates key trauma principles into the organizational culture" (SAMHSA Trauma and Justice Strategic Initiative, 2014, p. 9). McConnico and colleagues (2016) use the terms *trauma informed* and *trauma sensitive* interchangeably to describe a trauma-sensitive approach to education as encompassing policies and practices based in knowledge of trauma with the intent to build community, belonging, social justice, capacity, and resilience, and to avoid re-traumatization of children and parents.

While these more global descriptions of trauma-informed approaches and trauma-sensitive education are useful at an organizational level, there is a utility in considering these concepts for hands-on application in a clinical practice setting. To that end, we offer the following definitions which distinguish between the terms *trauma aware, trauma sensitive*, and *trauma informed*. *Trauma awareness* is something that most mental health professionals learn in their graduate school training. It is defined as a foundational awareness that trauma is widespread, covers a large range of adverse experiences, and that its impacts on people are as unique as each individual (Attachment & Trauma Network [ATN], 2024).

In contrast, *trauma sensitivity* includes a foundation of trauma awareness that involves learning and integrating specific skills, language, and practices in one's practice, whether or not a client has a trauma history

(Mindremapping Academy, 2023). *Trauma informed* is a more global approach aimed at developing organizations, communities, or institutions that foster recovery from trauma and avoid re-traumatization across all levels from clients, to practitioners, to support staff, to custodians and beyond (Mindremapping Academy, 2023).

Two other concepts are important for working in a trauma-sensitive manner: the zone of proximal development (Vygotsky, 1980) and the window of tolerance (Siegel, 1999). The zone of proximal development aligns with the concept of comfort zones that we discussed in Chapter 1. The zone of proximal development provides a different perspective than comfort zones that is especially useful in the context of addressing trauma. As an aside, even though we discuss the zone of proximal development in the context of trauma, all of us have zones of proximal development regardless of whether we have experienced trauma.

Vygotsky's (1980) zone of proximal development was meant to help educators understand the level of support or scaffolding a student needs to learn new content, examining what a student can do on their own, what they can do with help, and what they can't do. The scaffolding or support needed comes into focus for tasks a student "can do with help" and "what they can't do," and the educator provides supports or scaffolding to foster student learning so that a task that was labeled "can do with help" becomes a task they "can do on their own," and a task that was labeled "can't do" becomes a task they "can do with help" in an iterative way so that eventually the student can do all the tasks on their own (Vygotsky, 1980). A similar iterative process of scaffolding occurs in the Experiential Therapy settings. However, unlike education, where the teacher prepares the lessons and determines what supports are needed, in Experiential Therapy the clinician brings relevant Experiential Therapy activities, but the client is empowered to use challenge by choice and clinical segues to create the elements of their own scaffolding. In trauma-sensitive Experiential Therapy the iterative process is deepened as clients are empowered to understand and apply their own zone of proximal development as they use challenge by choice and the clinical segues.

In therapeutic settings the zone of proximal development gets translated into three zones: the safe zone, the challenge zone, and the overwhelmed zone (Germer & Neff, 2019). "The optimal zone for learning is in the *challenge* zone, which is between the comfort zone of feeling *safe* and the danger zone of being overwhelmed" (Germer & Neff, 2019, p. 100). In this way, the zone of proximal development overlaps quite nicely with the concept of the comfort zone and challenge by choice. In the trauma literature the challenge zone coincides with the window of tolerance (Siegel, 2012), which adds another foundational concept for trauma-sensitive Experiential Therapy. The window of tolerance expands our thinking about the challenge zone. Commonly, when clients are in the challenge zone, they are ready for the challenge or learning. However, the window of tolerance broadens our perspective: if clients are in their window of tolerance, then they are at the optimal place for learning within the challenge zone. However, if a client is in the challenge zone, but is moving out of their window of tolerance, then the aim is for them to move toward the safe zone.

The window of tolerance is a person's capacity to be psychologically and physically comfortable in the face of challenging stressors, emotions, thoughts, and/or physical experiences (Hershler, 2021; Siegel, 1999). Everyone, regardless of trauma history, has a window of tolerance. Some of us have wider windows and can handle more stressors while remaining comfortable, and others of us have narrower windows, meaning that we experience more discomfort in the face of stress, and our window of tolerance can change depending on the context we are in or over time (Emerson & Hopper, 2011). People with trauma histories tend to have narrower windows of tolerance and can easily become activated and find themselves unable to access strategies to manage suffering (Hershler, 2021). For trauma survivors, even "moderate emotions or physiological reactivity [can] become untenable and serve to activate traumatic memories" (Hershler, 2021, p. 25).

When a person is in their window of tolerance, they are able to be aware of their feelings, thoughts, and body sensations while simultaneously taking in pleasant, unpleasant, or neutral information and/or experiences (Hershler, 2021). For example, the client who is their window of tolerance can notice they have an unpleasant feeling or sensation in the pit of their stomach when they recall a traumatic memory and can use a breathing strategy, movement strategy, or cognitive strategy to release the unpleasant feeling and avoid being overwhelmed by it. That is, they don't push the unpleasant feeling or sensation away, but because they are in their window of tolerance they can process it in the moment with a breathing, movement, or cognitive strategy and can continue with whatever they were doing when the memory arose. In contrast, the person who is activated outside of their window of tolerance by the trauma memory may become hyper-aroused or hypo-aroused. When a person becomes hyper-aroused, they may react with a fight or flight reaction, experience an increased heart rate that might feel like panic, have feelings of anger, fear, or anxiety, experience their muscles becoming tense such as making tightly closed fists, or they might have thoughts of dread and worry that make them think "something bad is going to happen to me," "I have to get out of here," or "I'm in trouble" (Hershler, 2021, p. 26). When a person becomes hypo-aroused, they might experience feelings of "deep sadness, loneliness, or shame, their body may feel numb, heavy, sleepy or even disconnected and they may have thoughts such as 'why bother,' 'I'm tired,' 'something is wrong with me' and may even seek out a hiding place or go to sleep" (Hershler, 2021, p. 26).

A key point is that when someone is outside of their window of tolerance (hyper-aroused or hypo-aroused) they lose access to their social engagement system, which is our capacity to garner support from oneself or to access supportive people in our lives (Treleavan, 2018). "The social engagement system is intrinsically self-calming and is, therefore, built-in protection against one's own organism being 'hijacked' by the sympathetic arousal system [fight, flight] and/or frozen into submission by the more primitive emergency shutdown system" (Levine, 2010, p. 94). Our role as Experiential Therapy clinicians is to support clients in moving slowly and being empowered to become aware of their window of tolerance so they can develop skills that will allow them to widen it without veering into hyper- or hypo-arousal. The caution is that many clients will focus on striving or pushing themselves, and in group settings clients can get caught up in the energy of a group's excitement about an activity and dive full in before they are ready. However, pushing oneself or being pushed by others beyond the window of tolerance before they are ready can exacerbate trauma, make the window of tolerance smaller, and take clients outside of their capacity for self-regulation (Treleaven, 2018). Clinicians and client alike can build skills for supporting the process in a slow and iterative manner. These skills are discussed in the next sections.

Trauma Sensitivity: Skills for Clinicians

Emerson and Hopper (2011) are perhaps some of the earliest scholar-practitioners to bring trauma sensitivity practices and skills into focus through their development of trauma-sensitive yoga. While these practices and skills were developed in the context of yoga, many of them are applicable across modalities. We discuss language first. The general approach for trauma-sensitive language is an awareness that trauma survivors are often attuned to not only what is said, the words used, but also to *how* something is said (e.g., tone of voice) (Emerson & Hopper, 2011). In this sense, Emerson and Hopper (2011) suggest using a tone of voice and cadence that are perhaps slower than usual and that have a calming quality as a means to help clients develop the capacity to move slowly and to "experience each moment in time"

(p. 120). Another general aim of trauma-sensitive language is to use words that foster clients' development of interoceptive awareness in the present by not being directive as to where in the body clients might experience that awareness (Emerson & Hopper, 2011). For example, when introducing an experiential therapy activity, the clinician might say, *as I describe our next activity, be curious about how your body reacts, maybe you notice a sensation in it or maybe you don't, either way it is okay.* Or, *as we stand in this circle see what you notice about how you are standing and if you choose, you might make any adjustment that makes standing here feel more comfortable for you.* This kind of language can then be extended to support clients in noticing interoceptive awareness and thoughts and feelings that arise with body reactions during more intense Experiential Therapy activities. This fosters clients' awareness of somatic and other experiences in the context of each activity and can be a bridge for clients to ascertain a more concrete sense of whether they are in the safe zone, learning zone, or panic zone and to use that information when making a choice for challenge by choice. Emerson and Hopper (2011) refer to this kind of language as the *language of inquiry* (Emerson & Hopper, 2011). The language of inquiry is meant to empower clients to observe and to explore, and uses words and phrases such as "notice," "be curious," "approach with interest," "allow," and "experiment" (Emerson & Hopper, 2011, p. 120).

Trauma-sensitive practice is also meant to foster a context of nonjudgment either toward oneself or toward others. The idea is that each client is choosing to participate in any capacity, including standing back and observing, without fear of judgment. Of course, this is a common value and ethic across all therapeutic contexts and modalities. The trauma-sensitive piece comes into play with the use of invitational language, which is meant to verbally and directly foster choice, control, and empowerment with key phrases such as "as you are ready," "if you like" (Emerson & Hopper, 2011, p. 121), or "you're invited," "possibly," "perhaps," "if it feels available to you," "you may stop or pause at any time for any reason." For example, when introducing an Experiential Therapy activity, the clinician might say, *as you are ready, take one step toward the center of the circle; or you're invited to stay where you are now or to take as many steps toward the center of the circle as feels right for you; the choice is completely up to you.* One caveat related to invitational language is that clear and unambiguous directions are imperative to create and maintain safety (Emerson & Hopper, 2011). This is abundantly important in Experiential Therapy.

The next set of trauma-sensitive skills are observation skills for noticing hyper- and hypo-arousal in clients. We offer these skills with the caveat that clients' stress or overwhelm experiences might not aways be visible, so learn to be in good contact with clients to increase the chances that you are able to be aware if they move out of their zone of tolerance. Treleaven (2018) provides an excellent list of potential signs that a client may be leaving their zone of tolerance. These include muscle tone that is collapsed or muscle tone that is tight and tense, difficulty breathing, hyperventilation, sweating, jumping and startling at the slightest sound or movement, skin tone becoming shades lighter than usual (like the person has seen a ghost), emotional volatility such as rage, fierce anger or fierce fear, terror, sobbing with uncontrollable tears (Treleaven, 2018). Clinicians might also observe edginess, irritability, anxiety, and panic when clients are hyper-aroused and sadness, exhaustion, and isolating behaviors when clients are hypo-aroused (Grabbe & Miller-Karas, 2018). The key is that when you observe a client in hyper-arousal they may seem to want to fight or flee, and when you see clients in hypo-arousal they may seem like they want to shut down or freeze; however, these are not choices, this is their early warning system or autonomic nervous system, the sentry taking over and reacting to what feels like intense threat or danger (National Institute for the Clinical Application of Behavioral Medicine, 2019).

Trauma Sensitivity: Skills for Clients

We honor and empower our clients when we collaborate with them to develop tools for their own self-soothing and awareness. In this section we describe skills you can help clients learn that will enable them to work within their zone of tolerance. Since trauma is so widespread it makes the most sense to teach these skills to all of your clients, regardless of whether they disclose any trauma history. As we noted earlier in this chapter, everyone has a window of tolerance, and on some days the window can be wider or narrower than on others. Clients with trauma experiences just tend to have narrower windows of tolerance and are likely more vulnerable to moving quickly into hyper- or hypo-arousal when they become activated by trauma memory, either physical, emotional, cognitive, or environmental. Therefore these skills are applicable for all clients.

The first step involves educating all of your clients about the window of tolerance (Siegel, 2012). Experiential Therapy offers excellent opportunities for this because teaching about the window of tolerance goes hand in hand with teaching about the zone of proximal development and challenge by choice with the comfort zones of relax, learning, or panic. We encourage you to craft the lesson by using the information we provide in this chapter. Another excellent resource is *Looking at Trauma: A Tool Kit for Clinicians* (Vol. 23) (Hershler et al., 2021), which you can find in our reference list. There are additional resources you can use, such as the infographic about the window of tolerance developed specifically for clients by the National Institute of Clinical and

Behavioral Medicine (NICABM) (2019). We suggest using this as a handout that clients can take with them as NICABM offers it for anyone's use as long as they include the copyright information which is listed at the bottom of the infographic. NICABM offers more details about the window of tolerance at the following website: https://www.nicabm.com/trauma-how-to-help-your-clients-understand-their-window-of-tolerance/. Once your clients have knowledge of the window of tolerance (Siegel, 2012), you can teach them skills for assessing their window of tolerance and skills for putting on the brakes (Rothchild, 2011).

Assessing One's Own Window of Tolerance

Treleaven (2018) suggests using an arousal scale for clients to assess their level of arousal on a continuum from zero to 10 where ratings at the lower end of the scale represent hypo-arousal, ratings in the middle of the scale represent being in the window of tolerance, and ratings toward the high end of the scale represent hyper-arousal. In reality, it is less about the number that clients use to rate their window on any particular day and more about them getting a gauge of awareness each time they use the scale; therefore we do not suggest that you offer clients a range of what ratings might equate to being hypo-aroused, in the window, or hyper-aroused. If they request a frame of reference for the numbers, we encourage you to ask them to choose the rating that fits best. For example, if they reflect and notice they're feeling extremely tired, exhausted, lethargic, immobilized, then they may want to rate themselves toward the hypo-arousal end of the scale, choosing a number toward that end that they think best fits their level of these feelings (Treleaven, 2018). On the other hand, if they reflect that they are feeling extremely shook up, anxious, or panicky, they may want to rate themselves toward the hyper-arousal end of the scale, choosing a number toward that end that they think best fits their level of these feelings (Treleaven, 2018). If they reflect that they are feeling within their window of tolerance, that they are up for learning and engaging in challenge, then they may want to rate themselves toward the center of the scale. "While the actual numbers students and clients report are slightly arbitrary, using the scale enables them to track and determine their level of arousal, gives them an ongoing reference point about the breadth of their range, and enables them to self-report to teachers or clinicians on their level of internal arousal" (Treleaven, 2018, p. 109).

Whenever we use scales or other self-assessments such as this one, we find it helpful to create a handout to give clients a hands-on and visual image of the rating scale with numbers and words (see Treleaven, 2018, p. 109, for an example). The scale can be used in many ways, perhaps just before each Experiential Therapy activity begins, to help clients consider how they want to manage challenge by choice. Another option is to use the scales before and after each activity or at the beginning, middle, and end of the day. Additionally, when we are outside and do not have papers, we will use a simple thumb technique: thumb completely up means panic zone, thumb in the middle means learning zone, and thumb pointing down is in the relax zone.

Musheer (2021) developed a trigger scale that could dovetail quite nicely with the window of tolerance assessment. Musheer's scale (2021) directs clients to consider three different levels of being triggered as demonstrated by physical sensations, feelings, thoughts, or impulses. At the low end, clients might be experiencing all or any combination of "physical sensations (shortness of breath or holding their breath, tightness in the chest, numbness), feelings (anxiety, irritation, hurt) or thoughts (here we go again, it's happening again) or impulses (a desire to hide or leave and get away)" (Musheer, 2021, p. 30). At the medium level, clients might be experiencing all or any combination of "physical sensations (increased level of energy/tension or numbness in the body, heavy limbs, fogginess), feelings (fear, sadness, shame, anger), thoughts (this always happens to me, something is wrong with me, why bother?), impulses (to sleep, run, or yell)" (Musheer, 2021, p. 30). At the highest level, clients might be experiencing all or any combination of "physical sensations (significant energy/tension, uncontainable urgency, total numbness, reduced vision), feelings (rage, hopelessness, helplessness, worthlessness), thoughts (I'm not worth it, nothing is going to work, I don't want to live another day like this), impulses (to fight, hurt self or others, or collapse). (Musheer, 2021, p. 30).

Musheer (2021) provides some useful tips for talking with clients about the scale, suggesting that you begin in a general way by asking clients to share any ideas on experiences some might have in their body, feelings, thoughts, or actions when they get triggered or activated. This can facilitate a discussion about what can happen when someone is activated and perhaps how far out of their zone of tolerance they might go, depending on the trigger and what kinds of body sensations, feelings, thoughts, or actions might occur at different points from when someone is in their zone of tolerance compared to when someone is moving into hyper- or hypo-arousal. Beginning in a more general mode, considering how people in general experience triggers, allows clients to engage without having to reveal their own experiences before they are ready. This can be followed up by a more personal discussion with the client about their own experiences.

After getting clients to consider what trigger experiences might look like for others generally and for themselves more specifically, you can move into identifying triggers, once again in a more general way and then, if it seems clinically appropriate, you can move toward clients revealing things that they know trigger them (Musheer, 2021). After this, you can use the scale with clients so they can begin to assess their body, feeling, thought, and action responses to triggers. It is important to help clients understand that their reactions might fall across the scale such that they might have some body sensations at the low level of the scale, feeling reactions at the medium level, and thoughts at the high level (Musheer, 2021). Knowledge is power; the more familiar clients become with what triggers them and their different body, feeling, thought, and action responses, they can then begin to use that information to know when they need to step out of an activity in order to stay in their zone of tolerance or when they are ready to engage with challenge if they are more solidly within their window. This knowledge allows them to begin to get a sense of when they need to put on the brakes, as we discuss next.

Skills for Putting on the Brakes

Babette Rothschild (2011) created the concept of *putting on the brakes*, which is the idea that clients can slow the pace of their engagement and slow down, or put on the brakes, so they can stay within their window of tolerance. The Seeking Safety Curriculum (Najavits, 2002) offers some excellent and evidence-based grounding techniques that clients can use to return to their window of tolerance. Najavits (2002) describes exercises to promote mental grounding, physical grounding, and soothing grounding. We share some of these here with two caveats. One is that clients will only know to use these skills if they have first learned to identify when they are about to move toward the edges of their window, hence the importance of helping clients to use the zone of arousal scale (Treleaven, 2018) and the trigger scale (Musheer, 2021) we just described. The second caveat is that clients need to learn and practice the grounding skills many times so that when they are needed, they can call them up and easily apply them.

Najavits (2002) describes grounding as a strategy to disengage from emotional pain by turning one's focus outside of themselves toward some external experience. The strategies are subtle and not typically visible to others, so they can be used anytime and anywhere (Najavits, 2002). Najavits (2002) offers these guidelines: keep your eyes open and look around your location (e.g., room, store, street); avoid verbalizing or writing down negative emotions or thoughts because the aim is to get away from these feelings and thoughts; avoid judgments (e.g., if you are focused on three things that you can smell, just notice the smell and dismiss any thoughts that you like or dislike the scents); whichever strategy you choose, be in the present, not the past or the future. Grounding is not meant to be relaxing or relaxation training; instead, it is action oriented (Najavits, 2002). Next, we describe some of the grounding strategies.

One mental grounding strategy includes describing all of the elements of a room, such as the color of the walls, the number of windows, the furniture, the flooring, the temperature (Najavits, 2002). This also applies to describing any environment where you are located, including the outdoors. Another mental grounding strategy that is common is to notice 5 things you see, notice 4 things that you can touch, notice 3 things that you can hear, notice 2 things that you can smell, and notice one thing that you can taste. A third grounding strategy is to describe something you do every day in extreme detail (Najavits, 2002); this could be washing dishes, taking the train to work, or brushing your teeth.

One physical grounding strategy is to move your body and notice every movement while stretching, walking, or any other body movement (Najavits, 2002). Another physical grounding is to hold your hands under warm or cool water, whichever feels best (Najavits, 2002). A third physical grounding could include touching things around you, such as car keys or books, or even carrying a grounding object, such as a small stone or marble, in a pocket that you can reach for at any time.

Soothing grounding strategies include quietly saying positive things to yourself, such as *I am a good person having a difficult time and it is okay*; imagining pictures of supportive loved ones or friends; recalling the tune or lyrics to a soothing or favorite song (Najavits, 2002). In summary, it is key that clients choose or create the kind of grounding that works best for them and have several options in their back pocket in case one might work better depending on the circumstances. Clients will gravitate to different grounding strategies and may find one type more useful than another. The best way they can discover this is trying them out and practicing them before they need to use them.

Next Chapter

In the next chapter, we will discuss integrating mindfulness practices with Experiential Therapy.

Chapter 4
Integrating Mindfulness With Experiential Therapy

Mindfulness approaches take the stance that "problems are viewed as opportunities for growth" and encourage clients to understand problems as part of life, that life will always bring challenges, and the goal is to learn how to navigate them (Lee et al., 2009, p. 312). This stance pairs well with Experiential Therapy, which has the goal of learning through experience and applying that learning to the next challenges one will face.

Foundations of Mindfulness-Based Practices

Meditation and mindfulness and mind-body-spirit practices, such as yoga, tai chi, and qigong, originate from Buddhism, Hinduism, Daoism, Ayurveda, and both ancient and modern traditional Chinese medicine (Lee et al., 2009). These practices have been brought to the Western world in various ways, beginning as far back as the late 1800s when monks from India shared the practices and teachings of yoga with Western societies. More recently, the Dalai Lama's efforts to connect with practitioners and scholars at Emory University (https://tibet.emory.edu/) and with Richard Davidson, PhD, at the Center for Healthy Minds at the University of Wisconsin, Madison (https://www.centerhealthyminds.org/), represent another wave of intentionally sharing mind-body-spirit practices with the West. Thich Nhat Hanh, a Vietnamese Buddhist monk who passed in 2022, also played a large role in bringing mindfulness meditation to the West. His life and actions in that regard are honored in two recent documentaries about his life, *A Cloud Never Dies* and *I Have Arrived, I Am Home.* Thich Nhat Hanh has written over 100 books, such as *Peace Is Every Step*, *The Miracle of Mindfulness*, and *Silence, the Power of Quiet in a World Full of Noise*, that have fed the West's understanding and practice of mindfulness meditation and engaged Buddhism. Mina (2023) states that Thich Nhat Hanh "left a tremendous legacy as one of the major figures to bring mindfulness to the West and to expound

Understanding and Effectively Utilizing Experiential Therapy. Julie Anne Laser and Nicole Nicotera,
Oxford University Press. © Oxford University Press (2025). DOI: 10.1093/9780197757581.003.0004

the principles of engaged Buddhism as part of his own peace efforts during the Vietnam War" (Mina, 2023, para. 1).

When we use mind-body-spirit practices in our own work, it is of upmost importance and ethical practice to name and honor the traditions from which they arise. "It is imperative for practicing professionals to acknowledge the original source of the tradition [they are applying in their work]. . . . For instance, Ha breathing is based on the theory and practices of qigong . . . meditation practices and breathing exercises from Buddhism and Daoism" (Lee et al., 2009, p. 306). It is okay to adapt some practices and apply them in new ways; however, "it is unethical to use or modify techniques from other traditions without acknowledging the source or tradition" (Lee et al., 2009, p. 306). As an example, one of the authors attended a workshop that integrated neuroscience, mindfulness, and concepts related to moving away from self-focused ways of being to more interdependent ways of being as a means to promote well-being. The presenter closed the workshop with a series of slow, silent movements that they delivered as their own creation. Though the majority of the movements were recognizable as movements from qigong practices, the presenter did not name or honor the origins of these movements, which are from ancient and modern traditional Chinese medicine. This is considered cultural appropriation, and we ask you to avoid such errors. In this vein, if you choose to apply mindfulness, meditation, or other mind-body-spirit practices in your work, then develop and maintain a personal practice in which you use one or more mind-body-spirit practices, so you are aware of their sources of wisdom. Having your own practice will not only educate you about the sources of the practices, it will also allow you to facilitate mindfulness with clients from a more centered and knowing place.

What Is Mindfulness?

In an interview, Thich Nhat Hanh stated, "Mindfulness is when you are truly there, mind and body together. You breathe in and out mindfully, you bring your mind back to your body, and you are there. When your mind is there with your body, you are established in the present moment" (Nhat Hanh, 1997). Jon Kabat-Zinn (2013) defines mindfulness as being aware of your thoughts from moment to moment, without judging them or yourself, or getting caught up in the stories your thoughts are telling you. When we are mindful, we are not emptying our minds, nor are we stopping our minds from wandering (Kabat-Zinn, 2013). In fact, it is not possible to completely empty your mind of thoughts or to keep it from wandering (Jha, 2018). However, through the practice of mindfulness meditation we can develop the skill for focusing our minds and being aware of the present moment in our minds and bodies without judgment (Jha, 2018; Kabat-Zinn, 2013). The reason it is called a practice is that learning to bring your mind back to the present over and over again, without judgment, each time it wanders is a lifelong journey.

"Mindfulness is often described as a bell that reminds us to stop and silently listen" (Hanh, 2015, p. 4). What does it look like to stop and silently listen? Greenland (2012) provides a depiction to help people comprehend the skill of mindfulness or the capacity to stop and silently listen. She refers to this capacity as the ABCs of attention, balance, and compassion (Greenland, 2012). When we are in the attention mode, we become aware of what we are focused on, which is commonly more than one thing or even more than three things. With this awareness we can then choose which one thing to focus on in that moment. When we choose what to focus on, then we move to balance, which involves quieting the brain and seeing what we have chosen to focus on, noticing the thoughts, feelings, and body sensations that arise without trying to change them, regardless of whether they are pleasant, unpleasant, or neutral. Then we move to compassion, which involves caring and connecting, perhaps caring for our hearts if we noticed unpleasant thoughts, feelings, or body sensations, and connecting to a source of comfort, whether that is other people, a companion animal, or to ourselves by being our own best friend, offering a cup of tea for comfort.

The ABCs of attention, balance, and compassion (Greenland, 2012) can seem quite mysterious to clients who have not tried to practice mindfulness, so we suggest two tangible, hands-on ways to introduce them to the practice. We like to use scents or bubbles, depending on whether clients have allergies to scents. First, we describe using scents. We use two different essential oils and place them on cotton balls in different small plastic bags so that each client has two plastic bags, one for each scent. Then we ask them to use attention by opening one bag and focusing on the way it smells, and then to do the same with the other bag, focusing on each scent in the present moment. We teach some mindful breathing at this point, asking them to slowly inhale each scent through their nose and then asking then to slowly exhale through their nose three times for each scent. During this focusing we also ask them to notice how their mind wanders even as they smell each scent and that each time they notice their mind has wandered, to bring their attention back to the scent and their breath as they inhale and exhale. After this, we move to choosing and ask them to now choose to use only one of the scents or none of the scents, to notice how their mind may wander as they make the choice, but to bring their attention back to the scent and which one they want to choose or if they want to choose neither of the scents.

After they have chosen a scent or no scent, we move into balance, inviting them to engage in using their breath by slowly inhaling and slowly exhaling the scent they chose, or the air itself if they chose no scent, so they can quiet the brain and "see" the scent or the air itself through the "eyes" of their nose and notice their experience of it. Is it pleasant, unpleasant, or neutral, and might they be willing to allow whatever sensation they have to be present without trying to change it? For example, if they find themselves wishing they had chosen a different scent or wishing they had chosen no scent, we invite them to be with the choice they made, instead of getting wrapped up in wishing they had made a different choice. We invite them to continue to notice when their mind has wandered from the scent or the air itself and to bring it back to quieting and "seeing" the scent or the air itself, slowly inhaling and exhaling.

After working through balance, we move into compassion, or the caring and connecting part of the exercise. Here we invite them to connect with where the scent came from, what kind of plant, where might it have been grown, who grew it and harvested it, how did it get into the bottle and then to be here in their hands. Or, if they chose no scent at all, we invite them to connect with the air itself; if it has scent, where did it come from; if the air has no scent, how is it that the air is so pure there is no scent, how do we get pure air or scented air? We close by asking them to move into caring, by considering what kind of thanks or gratitude they can send for how the scent got here to be in their hands today, or how the air is full of its own scent or no scent at all.

The other exercise we use to introduce clients to the ABCs of attention, balance, and compassion (Greenland, 2012) involves the use of bubbles. As a caution, if you are working with a group, bubbles can create high energy, even in adult graduate students, as we have seen with our own students. So be prepared to use a lot of group-management skills and help the clients process how anticipation can make finding attention, balance, and compassion more complex.

We provide a container of bubbles for each client, and before we hand them out, we instruct them to not open the container when they get it, but to let it sit there in front of them or to hold it in their hands while they wait for more instructions. Then we begin with the attention part of the exercise and ask clients to focus their attention on the bottle of bubbles in front of them or in their hands while they slowly inhale and exhale as they prepare to make a choice to open it if they want to use the bubbles, or leave it closed if they want to observe others using the bubbles. We teach some mindful breathing at this point, asking them to slowly inhale through their nose and then slowly exhale through their nose three times as they focus on the container of bubbles and to notice how their mind wanders away from the bubble container to other things, but to use the sight or feel of the bubble container to bring their focus back to the choice at hand. Now that they are focused, we invite them to choose to either open the bubbles or leave them closed, with the instruction that if they open the bubbles to wait for the next instruction before removing the wand inside and blowing bubbles. Next, we invite them to choose how they want to use their breath to blow bubbles. We ask them to notice what they see, a lot of bubbles all at once, or bubbles moving alone and slowly. If they chose to observe how others use the bubbles, look to see how the bubbles come out of the wands of others around you, and see if you can match your exhales to when you see bubbles leaving a wand and inhale when you don't see bubbles in the air.

Next, we move into the balance part of the exercise, the quieting and seeing. We invite clients to quiet their brain and to use their breath by slowly inhaling and slowly exhaling so that if they chose to open the bubbles then, they see bubbles form on their exhale, or if they chose to not open the bubbles to notice the sensation of their breath as it leaves their nose. Whichever they chose, we invite them to "see" the effects of their choice by noticing any thoughts, feelings, or body sensations that arise. Are they pleasant, unpleasant, or neutral, and might they be willing to allow whatever sensation they have to be present without trying to change it? For example, if they find themselves wishing they had chosen to open the bubbles, or wishing they had chosen to not open the bubbles, can they be with the choice they made, instead of getting wrapped up in wishing they had made a different choice? We invite them to continue to notice when their mind has wandered from the bubbles, or their breath itself if they chose to keep the bubbles closed, to bring it back to quieting and "seeing" their choice as they slowly inhale and exhale.

Now we begin the compassion part of the exercise, the connecting and caring. First, we invite them to connect with where the bubbles came from; how did the liquid get into the bottle and then to be here in your hands, or the hands of others in the group if you chose to not open the bubbles? What workers made it possible for the bubbles to be in the container, and how did the containers get to the store where they were sold? What kind of thanks can you send to how the bubbles got here to be in your hands today?

Different Approaches to Mindfulness Practices

Many people have the misconception that mindfulness practices require a person to sit on a cushion, close their eyes, and be very still and silent for long periods of time. Fortunately, this is not at all the case. Mindfulness practices cover a continuum of actions, from more active and kinesthetic, such as yoga, to less active and intangible, such as sitting with the eyes closed and following the breath. Mindfulness can involve walking, standing, movement, smelling, seeing, touching, tasting, listening, singing, or chanting, as well as the traditional view many people have in which someone sits still and quietly on a cushion with their eyes closed. Additionally, a mindful practice could take place for one or two minutes while driving in traffic, or take place for 45 minutes of a yoga or qigong practice, or take place for longer periods of sitting silently. It is up to each individual to find and practice mindfulness in a way that best supports their needs, which may change over time.

As Experiential Therapy clinicians, we are commonly in a position to bring or suggest mindfulness exercises during a session. Pollack and colleagues (2014) provide a wonderful guide for considering what kind of practice might be most supportive depending on how distracted or settled a client's mind, body, or spirit is. If clients are more distracted, then practices that engage the body, such as walking or standing, are useful as this could involve a focus on the feel of the feet or hands on a surface, taking in the sights or sounds of nature, or eating meditation (Pollack et al., 2014). When clients are more settled, then you might use subtler practices such as silently repeating a *gatha* or *mantra*, or focusing on the breath in the belly, or even subtler noticing the breath as it enters and leaves the nose (Pollack et al., 2014).

Your role, as the clinician, is to check in with clients and use your observational skills to assess where they are on the continuum of distracted to settled. Therefore, it is key to have an array of mindfulness tools in your back pocket so you can choose whatever might best support the needs of your clients on any given day. Having your own regular mindfulness practice is also imperative as it not only will help you understand how you are impacted by different practices when you are more distracted or more settled, but also will build your capacity for combining elements that can accommodate groups of clients who will most likely be presenting on various places in the distracted to settled continuum.

Focused attention and open monitoring are two broad categories of mindfulness practice that can serve a useful tool in the context of supporting clients who are in different places on the distracted to settled continuum. Focus attention and open monitoring are the main mediation skills within Buddhist meditation practices (Lutz et al., 2008). Focused attention mindfulness or meditation (FAM) "is a concentrative practice with a well-defined target object such as the breath sensation. Meditators repeatedly focus and maintain their attention on the target object avoiding distractions from internal (e.g., thought) or external (e.g., sounds) sources" (Yoshida et al., 2020, p. 216). Open monitoring mindfulness or meditation (OMM) "is a practice that focuses on staying in the nonreactive monitoring state without defining the target object. Meditators monitor the content of experience (e.g., bodily sensations, feelings and thoughts) from moment to moment with nonreactive and non-judgmental awareness" (Yoshida et al., 2020, p. 216). FAM is a foundational practice through which people develop skills for managing and monitoring their attention and is viewed as a building block for the capacity to practice OMM skills (Lutz et al., 2008).

FAM is more structured, and clients follow a series of steps that they actively attempt to complete (Waelde, 2022). An example of this could be as concrete as an eating or beverage meditation in which clients are facilitated in following a sequence of steps to engage the mind and body in contemplative eating or drinking a beverage such as tea or coffee. An eating or beverage mediation can be done more formally for a specific period while sitting, or more informally such as for the first part of a meal. There is a wonderful eating and a wonderful tea/coffee meditation available on the Plum Village App, which is associated with Thich Nhat Hanh's monastery in France.

On the other hand, FAM could be less concrete than an eating or beverage meditation during which clients follow a *gatha*, or sequence of phrases that they silently repeat to themselves in combination with inhaling and exhaling. Thich Nhat Hanh's teachings offer many *gatha*s, such as the following one which can be silently recited in its entirety or shortened to one word for each inhale and exhale. It can be done while walking, standing, sitting, or lying down and can be practiced more formally for a set period or more informally at any moment, such as while doing the dishes or standing in line at the store:

Breathing in, I know I am breathing in. Breathing out, I know I am breathing out (In. Out.). Breathing in, my breath grows deep. Breathing out, my breath grows slow (Deep. Slow.). Breathing in, I'm aware of my body. Breathing out, I calm my body (Aware of body. Calming.) Breathing in, I smile. Breathing out, I release. (Smile. Release.) Breathing in, I dwell in the present moment. Breathing out, I enjoy the present moment. (Present moment. Enjoy.) (Hanh, 2015, p. 43)

In contrast to FAM, OMM is not structured. Instead, the person meditates more freely and "is open to perceive and observe any sensation or thought without focusing on a concept in the mind or a fixed item; therefore, attention is flexible and unrestricted" (Colzato et al., 2012, p. 116). The person does not attempt to focus on anything specific, nor do they try to keep any awareness of experience at bay. In essence, the aim is to be in the present and keep coming back to the present as you notice your thoughts have drifted to past or the future. Each time you notice and return to your present experience of "being" is a moment of pure mindfulness, open awareness.

An OMM could involve using a meditation timer, such as the Insight Timer, or simply the timer on a cell phone, and setting it for a period, however long feels most supportive. When the timer starts, take a meditation posture, which is meant to help a person be grounded and centered in their body and in an upright, but not uptight position, so there is room for their lungs to breathe in and out, yet also a space for the body to have relaxed attention. The following directions might be helpful. Begin with grounding and centering: (1) find a quiet and comfortable place to sit; (2) notice the places where your body meets the surface you are sitting on, notice your feet on the earth and allow your head to gently lift toward the sky; (3) inhale and raise your shoulders toward your ears and when you exhale gently lower your shoulder away from your ears three times; (4) lower your gaze to one small point on the ground in front of you, or if it feels supportive, close your eyes and continue to slowly and comfortably inhale and exhale. Now you are ready to being OMM meditation by following one instruction and practice for as little as one minute or are much as 30 minutes or more, after you have set up your meditation posture. One useful instruction is from Healthy Minds Innovations, which is associated with the Center for Healthy Minds at the University of Wisconsin:

> The practice here is to be aware, but not to direct attention or control your experience in any way. If you're aware, that's it. There is nothing more to do. For the next minute or so let go of control and simply be present. If your attention moves around, let it. If thoughts come and go, don't worry. Just let them come and go freely. It'll probably be challenging to stay present and aware; that's normal. When you notice you've been lost, you don't have to do anything extra. The moment you're back in the present moment, just let go and rest in that state of awareness. (Healthy Minds Innovations, n.d., sound cloud recording)

It can be helpful to use a timer that will ring a bell or a tone every minute so that your wandering mind has a reminder to come back to the present moment awareness.

We hope you now have a good idea of the difference between FAM meditation and OMM meditation. We direct you back to the continuum we discussed, with distractedness at one end and settled at the other. Now make the connection between using FAM exercises when clients are more distracted and the possibility of using more OMM exercises if a client is more settled. One important caveat is that when clients are emotionally dysregulated, even if they seem settled, you will want to use FAM exercises (Waelde, 2022).

How Do Mindfulness Practices Support Healing and Recovery?

The regular practice of mindfulness meditation helps us to access within ourselves the openhearted spaciousness characteristic of pure awareness and to express it in how we act in the world. Mindfulness as a regular practice can literally and figuratively give your life back to you, especially if you are stressed or in pain, or caught up in uncertainty and emotional turmoil—which of course, we all are to one degree or another in some moments or times in our lives. (Kabat-Zinn, 2021, p. 785)

There is growing evidence that supports the positive effects of regular mindfulness and meditation practices, for general well-being as well as for healing and recovery. The caveat is that the evidence suggests that having a regular mindfulness mediation practice is what leads to the benefits. Mindfulness meditation is not a magic pill that can be taken in any moment to make one's internal or external life better or even less stressful; it is not like taking an aspirin when you have a headache (Kabat-Zinn, 2021). Instead, as Jon Kabat-Zinn (2021) points out, a regular practice or either informal or formal mediation, whatever shape that takes for each individual, is needed to fully reap the benefits.

Studies from neuroscience indicate that a regular mindfulness meditation practice can promote the capacity for regulating emotions, which plays a role in being able to handle stress and reactivity (Kral et al., 2018). Mindfulness practices are also associated with perceived stress (Feng et al., 2019), as well as coping with stress and self-regulation (Leitch, 2017). In one study, 11 weeks of participating in mindfulness-skills training demonstrated stronger capacity for distress tolerance in medical students (Kraemer et al., 2016), while 6 weeks of a course of mindfulness-based self-care demonstrated reductions of burnout in social work graduate students (Maddock et al., 2021). Compassion meditation practice has been shown to reduce depression scores in adults, and a regular mindful meditation group was associated with increases in emotional stability and responses to stress (Desbordes et al., 2012). Compassion meditation has also been associated with increased life satisfaction, reductions in anxiety, reductions in depression, as well as the capacity to manage emotionally painful thoughts and feelings as opposed to fusing with them (Kyeong, 2013; Neff, 2003; Neff & Germer, 2013). Six weeks of a course in mindfulness-meditation skills and practice resulted in lowered rates of perceived stress, improved sleep quality, and capacity for self-compassion (Greeson, 2014; Rogers & Maytan, 2019).

While the science for mindfulness with youth is still quite young, there is evidence that it is protective for depression and self-esteem in Latinx queer youth managing bias-based victimization at school (Toomey & Anhalt, 2016). Mindfulness practice has also been associated with increasing self-compassion and reducing stress and depression in Latinx youth (Edwards et al., 2014). In another study, mindfulness practices were shown to reduce perceptions of stress and stress biomarkers (e.g., cortisol levels) in Native Hawaiian/Pacific Islander youth (Le & Proulx, 2015). A regular yoga and mindfulness practice conducted within an elementary school demonstrated reductions in rumination, intrusive thoughts, and emotional arousal (Mendelson et al., 2010).

Mindfulness practices are also associated with the ability to expand the window of tolerance because they engage people in acquiring skills for somatic or interoceptive awareness so that individuals can employ more useful responses to perceived and real threats, rather than becoming mired in the reactivity of hypo- or hyper-arousal (Emerson & Hopper, 2011; Ford & Hawke, 2012; Leitch et al., 2009; Levine, 1997; Ogden et al., 2006; van der Kolk et al.; 2014; Warner et al., 2014). These enhanced skills for interoception and expanding the window of tolerance are important for all the clients you will serve and especially important for your clients who have experienced trauma.

Mindfulness and Trauma

A key thing to keep in mind as you read this chapter is that "mindfulness doesn't cause trauma—it's the practice of mindfulness meditation, offered without an understanding of trauma, that can exacerbate and entrench traumatic symptoms" (Treleaven, 2018, p. xxv). You already have an understanding of trauma and trauma sensitivity from reading Chapter 3, where we discussed trauma, trauma sensitivity, and skills for helping clients assess their window of tolerance. We refer you back to that content to review all those important details before you embark on integrating trauma sensitivity into your Experiential Therapy practice. This section of Chapter 4 will add to the knowledge you gained from Chapter 3 so you can carefully integrate mindfulness into Experiential Therapy activities with clients who have experienced trauma.

Mindfulness, as we defined it earlier, is paying attention to the present moment over and over again without judgment to build awareness of thoughts, feelings, and body sensations as they arise. The problem that can occur for people who have experienced trauma is that the experience lives in their body, mind, and spirit, and these experiences are more than likely to arise during mindfulness practices (Treleaven, 2018). Before you consider adding mindfulness to your Experiential Therapy practice, we highly recommend teaching your clients, whether or not they report a history of trauma, about the window of tolerance and assessing their own window of tolerance. We also highly recommend that you ask clients if they have a mindfulness meditation practice as part of your assessment, including what kind of mindfulness they practice (e.g., yoga, qigong, walking meditation, sitting meditation), how often they practice, and what it is like for them to practice. Then when you incorporate mindfulness practices into Experiential Therapy activities, we also highly recommend that you first teach clients to use the "seeking safety" activities we discussed in Chapter 3, and second, that you choose practices that engage the more structured experience of FAM as opposed to OMM, as discussed earlier in this chapter.

Waelde (2022) provides several mindfulness practices assessment questions you can use with clients. As a general guide, she suggests that if clients report having current or past mindfulness practice that you ask them to share the type of practice and if they used it as part of other therapy or if they used it on their own (Waelde, 2022). More specifically, Waelde (2022) suggests using these questions:

(1) Do you currently have a mindfulness mediation (MM) practice? (2) How often do you practice MM? Is your practice primarily in daily life? Do you practice sitting meditation? How often? Do you practice with a group, a mobile app, or primarily on your own? (3) What type of MM practice do you do? (4) What has been your response to MM? Has it been helpful? Are there things about MM that are especially difficult? (5) What are your views and expectations of MM for stress and trauma? (p. 79)

If some clients do not have any experience with MM, that is okay, as none is required (Waelde, 2022). Another important gauge the answers to these questions will provide is if a client is opposed to MM on either personal or religious grounds.

The books and mobile apps on mindfulness meditation are widespread, and if you choose to integrate mindfulness into your Experiential Therapy practice, we direct you a few here so you can first build your own practice if you do not have one, and then second, choose from the many different ideas and options available. We just maintain that you use focused attention practices more than open monitoring as a cautious approach that will take unknown trauma into account. We repeat several books by Thich Nhat Hanh that we mentioned earlier in this chapter: *Peace Is Every Step*, *The Miracle of Mindfulness*, and *Silence, the Power of Quiet in a World Full of Noise*. We also suggest Brenda Salgado's *Real-World Mindfulness for Beginners: Navigate Daily Life One Practice at a Time* and Jon Kabat-Zinn's *Wherever You Go, There You Are: Mindfulness Meditation in Everyday Life*.

Mindfulness Practices in the Context of Experiential Therapy

In summary, pairing Experiential Therapy with Mindfulness practices further increases the depth and breadth of the experience. Mindfulness brings clients into present moment awareness of the Experiential Therapy activity itself, so they are totally engaged in the present moment of the activity and the feelings, thoughts, and body sensations that arise during it. Mindfulness interventions help people to regulate the automatic fight, flight, freeze responses of the nervous system (Marchand, 2014) and to build the capacity to regulate the challenges of trauma histories (Leitch, 2017). In other words, pairing mindfulness practices with Experiential Therapy fosters clients' ability to recognize when they are nearing the panic zone or leaving their window of tolerance and skillfully manage the experience so they can more successfully engage with the therapy process and bring themselves into the learning zone or relax zone, depending on what they need in that moment. While the use of a mindfulness practice during an Experiential Therapy activity has the capacity to enhance the client's experience and awareness, they would need to develop a mindfulness practice that works for them on a regular basis in order for them to reap the full benefits in their daily lives.

Next Chapter

In Chapter 5 we will discuss fine-tuning for the clinician in terms of their capacities for well-being and working across identities.

Chapter 5
Fine-Tuning for the Clinician

Capacities for Well-Being and Working Across Identities

There are two aspects of being a mental health clinician that are always present and always challenging. One of these is therapist well-being and active strategies for self-care. The other aspect is clinician fine-tuning to build the capacity for working across client identities, especially clients with minoritized identities. This chapter addresses both of these aspects with a view to the necessity of lifelong learning and growth in both areas.

Even though we know it is important, mental health clinicians and students in training to become therapists commonly let their own well-being and self-care habits slide. This chapter begins with content to help you consider the components of well-being and strategies for supporting your well-being, or what we call self-care-communities of care. After this, the chapter covers content on what you, as the therapist, can become aware of, learn and unlearn, so you can work respectfully with clients with multiple identities. Many people tend to think of this capacity to work respectfully across identities as bound up in recipes, such as what to do when working with people of color, or what to do when working with women, or what to do when working with gay couples. Our stance is different from this; we see working across identities as something for which the clinician prepares their mind and heart. This stance promotes the acknowledgment by practitioners of the social conditioning they have received from living in a society and world with oppressive perspectives and actions that cause harm toward people with minoritized identities and then unlearning these perspectives and actions to work respectfully across identities.

What Is Well-Being?

Well-being is a complex concept that often gets simplified to mean the presence of health or the absence of illness. In fact, well-being is the experience of health and the experience of illness and many things in-between because

Understanding and Effectively Utilizing Experiential Therapy. Julie Anne Laser and Nicole Nicotera,
Oxford University Press. © Oxford University Press (2025). DOI: 10.1093/9780197757581.003.0005

well-being is a dynamic process. A while ago, one of the authors wrote the following blog that we use here to help you consider well-being from an expanded and more dynamic view:

> Well-being has become a popular concept, but what does it really mean? Many people think of well-being and illness as polar opposites, that is, when they are ill then there is not an ounce of well-being in their bodies and when they are well there is an absence of illness. However, well-being is not an "either-or" condition. Instead, well-being can be defined as a holistic experience of balance in the face of imbalance that includes the body, mind, heart, and spirit. This holistic view helps us to remember that well-being is a condition of balance in our lives—moment by moment, day by day, and year by year as we weave together our experiences of strenuous hills, steady flat paths, and glorious, thrilling rides. Well-being incorporates all of these ups, downs, and flat paths, recognizing that our lives are not about perfection—but instead about integrating our capacities and strengths with our follies and foibles.
>
> Well-being is the idea that we can have the flu and feel physically depleted while at the same notice love in our hearts and peace in our minds. The key word in this is "notice," because when we have the flu our whole attention tends to focus on or notice that experience at the expense of noticing other aspects of our well-being and this makes our suffering from the flu more potent.
>
> The same idea of balance applies to the glorious, thrilling rides in life—when we're on that ride we want to hold on to it forever—forgetting that this ride is balanced with the steady, mundane, flat paths and the strenuous uphill journeys. Then when the glorious, thrilling ride reaches the flat lands or even stops short at a strenuous hill, we are dismayed and may wonder, what do I need to do differently next time to hold on to that glorious ride, "what is wrong with me" that I am back on the mundane path or exerting up this strenuous hill again?
>
> Well-being is the acceptance that life is a balance of the glorious rides, steady paths, and strenuous hills. It is accepting that each of us is the sum total of our strengths and our foibles, that our strengths do not disappear when we blunder, and our foibles do not disappear when we succeed. In this way, well-being is multifaceted, reminding us that wellness involves body, mind, heart, and spirit in an ever-shifting balance across experiences of glorious rides, flat paths, and strenuous hills. Well-being involves the capacity to notice and accept the multifaceted aspects of our lives, without trying to hold on to or push away any of the experiences. (Nicotera & Laser, 2019, para. 1–3)

This perspective on well-being can seem a bit ambiguous, so we share the work of Richard Davidson of the Center for Healthy Minds, who provides a useful container for thinking about well-being in his discussion of the four pillars of well-being, which he labels as awareness, connection, insight, and purpose in life (cited in Feldscher, 2018). Awareness is described as a person's capacity to attend to the present moment and themselves (body, mind, spirit) in that moment and to be able to focus on one thing at a time (Dahl et al., 2020). In an interview, Dr. Davidson suggested that an absence of focus and present moment awareness is rampant due to numerous technology tools, such as smart phones, in our hands all day long. He stated, "If your mind is distracted, it exacts a toll on your well-being," and he noted evidence from one study that 47% of U.S. adults are acting without paying attention to what they are doing, and that in fact those in the study described decreased happiness when they were distracted from the present moment (Feldscher, 2018, para. 7).

Fostering the pillar of awareness does not mean that we all need to get rid of our smart phones and other devices; instead, it shines a light on how important it is to take technology breaks and to focus on one thing at a time. We often think we can multitask, for example, respond to a text while listening to a lecture. However, multitasking is a myth. As Kate Jones states, "For things that require our conscious effort and concentration, it is all but impossible to do two things at once. People often assume (or pretend) that they are multitasking, but they are task-switching" (Jones, 2023, para. 4). She goes on to point out that mistakes are common when people are task-switching and that in a research study where people were required to multitask, they reported increased rates of stress and frustration and experienced more pressure (Mark et al., 2008).

Feldscher (2018) shares that Dr. Davidson states, "Connection refers to emotions that underpin successful relationships with others—kindness, empathy, and maintaining a positive outlook" (Feldscher, 2018, para. 10). We can think of connection as a feeling of caring for others, combined with the capacity to see the positive qualities in others and to view their contributions as beneficial (Dahl et al., 2020). It makes sense that this second pillar of well-being follows awareness, because to truly make connection with others we need to be in the present moment and aware of ourselves and them, as opposed to distracted. We can support our connection pillar of well-being by making dedicated time to talk with others, share moments of beauty with others, and offer appreciation for the presence of our families, friends, and communities (Dahl et al., 2020).

"Insight refers to self-knowledge concerning the manner in which emotions, thoughts, beliefs, and other factors are shaping one's subjective experience, and especially one's sense of self" (Dahl et al., 2020, p. 32201). In other words, insight promotes a person's capacity to be aware of and to refute negative self-talk or the judgmental stories we all are at risk of telling ourselves on a bad day (Dahl et al., 2020). Insight also promotes resilience, the capacity to promptly turn around and make a comeback from negative experiences (Dahl et al., 2020). The key is that not all experiences of insight are positive; for example, without guidance we might get lost in plenty of insight on what we did wrong in a particular situation and ruminate ourselves into a worse day than it was before we tried insight (Dahl et al., 2020). "For example, when experiencing an anxious thought, insight would enable one to recognize how one's fearful expectations are being shaped by memories and self-critical thoughts and are thus overly focused on negative outcomes. With diminished insight, one would accept these expectations and thoughts as reality, with little understanding of the factors that are influencing one's perception" (Dahl et al., 2020, p. 32,201). As such, we want to learn how to use insight in a balanced way so that we accept and learn from our foibles, but not get buried in them. We can then move from our foibles to forgive ourselves for being imperfect humans. Some people practice elements of cognitive behavioral therapy to promote a balanced insight; others may choose meditation. However, whichever you choose, be sure to have a good mentor and sounding board to support your process.

The fourth pillar of well-being is purpose in life, which "refers to a sense of clarity concerning personally meaningful aims and values that one is able to apply in daily life" (Dahl et al., 2020, p. 32,202). Dahl and colleagues (2020) suggest that all of our aims are linked to our values. They differentiate between *long-term aims*, from which we gain our aspirations that guide choices we make and actions we take over the long haul of our lives, and *shorter-term aims*, which might be about daily goals or goals that may take a year or two, such as earning a graduate degree. Regardless, the authors state that our aims give us purpose and meaning in life, which is essential for well-being (Dahl et al., 2020).

What Is Self-Care?

We view self-care as the building blocks of well-being, and we define it as "the purposeful actions people and organizations take that contribute to wellness and stress reduction" (Bloomquist et al., 2015, p. 293). We view self-care as expanded beyond the individual to include numerous aspects that foster well-being, including care for the physical body, our emotional and mental health, our social-community collective health, our spiritual health, our economic or financial health, and the health of the organizations where we work and play. In our view, self-care must include the notion of community of care, or the collective nature of how our capacity to self-care is bound up with communities. This is one of the important things that living through the COVID-19 pandemic has taught us: our well-being is interconnected with both the known and unknown people in our lives and those who are near to us and those who live across the globe.

The key to self-care is to ignore the popular notions that self-care is somehow an escape from one's life, that all one needs is an expensive spa day to promote their well-being. Instead, we echo the following quote "True self-care is not bath salts and chocolate cake, it's making the choice to build a life you don't need to escape from" (Wiest, n.d.). We encourage each of you to build lives that you want to be in and not ones you want to escape. Quite a few years ago, one of my colleagues, who shall remain nameless, was extremely exhausted from work, family, and life, and mentioned in passing, "I was wishing I'd have a car accident so I could spend time in the hospital and get some rest." I recall we remarked on what a warped perspective that was. We want you to find the self-care and communities of care that work for you, so you don't find yourself expressing a similar sentiment.

What each person does for self-care/community of care is unique and we would be remiss to suggest that we have the answers that will work for you. However, we do present some options that arise from research on strategies that have demonstrated efficacy for promoting well-being among helping professionals, such mental health clinicians.

Therapists who take time with their families, have an active hobby, or travel for pleasure were found to have reduced rates of compassion fatigue (Eastwood & Ecklund, 2008). Helping professionals who viewed the organization or workplace in a positive light also reported lower levels of compassion fatigue (Thompson et al., 2014).

Compassion fatigue has two elements: burnout and secondary traumatic stress (Stamm, 2009–2012). Stamm (2009–2012) points out that a clinician who experiences compassion fatigue may notice aspects of burnout alone, aspects of secondary traumatic stress alone, or a combination of both. *Burnout* "is associated with feelings of hopelessness and difficulties in dealing with work or in doing your job effectively. These negative feelings usually have a gradual onset. They can reflect the feeling that your efforts make no difference, or they can be associated with a very high workload or a non-supportive work environment" (Stamm, 2009–2012, p. 2). In contrast, *secondary trauma stress* (STS) occurs from "secondary exposure to extremely or traumatically stressful events [in your work with clients]. . . . The symptoms of STS are usually rapid in onset and associated with a particular event. They may include being afraid, having difficulty sleeping, having images of the upsetting event pop into your mind, or avoiding things that remind you of the event" (Stamm, 2009–2012, p. 2).

Helping professionals such as hospice workers who used self-care techniques such as emotional support, having a sense of spirituality, or having work-life balance reported enhanced levels of compassion satisfaction (Alkema et al., 2008). *Compassion satisfaction* manifests as the gratification you draw from your work with clients as a mental health clinician. It has been described as "a sense of fulfillment derived from seeing clients suffer less and watching them transform from the role of victim to survivor" (Radey & Figley, 2007, p. 208). When you experience compassion satisfaction, you may notice that you get joy out of assisting others, and you may have a positive sense about what you can offer to your clients, colleagues, the agency where you work, or beyond (Stamm, 2009–2012).

Compassion satisfaction, compassion fatigue, and burnout are commonly combined into what is called professional quality of life (Stamm, 2010). Evidence suggests that clinicians who use self-care strategies that help them to cope, to be social and interact with others, who have creative outlets, and who attend to their body or physical self-care showed enhanced rates of overall quality of life (Lawson & Myers, 2011), while therapists who have a capacity for mindfulness demonstrated improved levels of overall quality of life (Harker et al., 2016; Thomas, 2012; Thomas & Otis, 2010; Thompson et al., 2014; Thieleman & Cacciatore, 2014). An array of other researchers also suggest that mindfulness practices are an important ingredient in practitioner quality of life (Beck, 2016, 2020; Dalphon, 2019; Grise-Owens et al., 2016; Lay, 2016; Lee, 2020; Warren & Deckert, 2020). For those who do not have a mindfulness or meditation practice, the idea that it could have such a widespread impact on quality of life may seem like magic. However, there are neuroscientific reasons and evidence demonstrating that mindfulness and meditation promote emotion regulation, which is a major ingredient in handling reactivity to life and work stresses (Kral et al., 2018).

In summary, practicing self-care/community of care is like any other skill. You need to practice it and develop it into a habit so that if you were to skip a day it would feel the same as if you skipped a day of brushing your teeth. You may recall as a child how difficult it was to develop the habit of brushing your teeth. Developing and maintaining habits for self-care/community of care can be just as difficult. Therefore, we encourage you to start small and to build the habits that support your well-being to coincide with other things that are already habits in your life. For example, if you want to practice the self-care/community of care habit of putting your smart phone or other devices away for 30 minutes each day, then build that into something else you are already doing, such as drinking your morning cup of tea or coffee, so it won't feel like such a loss to let your devices be in a different room from you for 30 minutes.

Clinician Fine-Tuning for Working Across Identities

To bring the power of Experiential Therapy activities to clients with diverse and multiple identities, you need to fine-tune yourself. This means educating yourself to unlearn oppressive stereotypes and actions so you can respectfully work across identities. We discuss several areas to help you begin to think about how to fine-tune yourself and be on the lifelong journey of moving toward inclusive ways of being and interacting. We begin with the idea of mindset as a foundation for the journey. Then, we discuss educating yourself for historical and contemporary contexts of oppression. This is followed by a final section on avoiding oppressive curiosities.

Mindset

The idea of mindset serves as a foundation for what we like to think of as a lifelong journey of unlearning, learning, and growing. Mindset can be defined as a way of looking at the world, and each of our mindsets is a product of many things, including where we grew up, the cultures of our families and communities, the schools we attended, the life adventures and misadventures we have experienced. The beauty of mindset is that it is changeable, and we are the ones who can change it if we choose. When we talk about mindset in the context of fine-tuning the self to work across identities, we suggest that it means developing an awareness of and educating yourself about the biases, judgments, stereotypes, and stories you have been taught about people based on what they look like, how they present, or the identities they share with you.

We focus on the work of Dweck (2007), who has researched and written about what she labels a growth mindset. The growth mindset has several qualities that include: an openness to learning new things; the capacity to rise to challenges and even seek them out; a willingness to keep trying even when things get hard or you feel discouraged; belief that effort is the pathway toward building capacity and that constructive critique is a source of information for growth; and an attitude of graciousness toward others' successes (Dweck, 2007).

We recognize that each person reading this chapter has multiple identities. Some of these identities might create ease in your life because they mirror identities that hold unearned power and privilege in society, such as being white, male presenting, or heterosexual. Some of your identities may create struggle and harm in your life because they mirror identities that have been systematically oppressed. As you read, please try to account for all of your multiple identities. Try to be aware that you will likely feel uncomfortable when you face one of your privileged identities and consider how you benefit from historical and contemporary injustices. Try to stay in the growth mindset and remember that discomfort due to awareness of a privileged identity is not oppression, it is just discomfort. Additionally, as you read, you may become activated in the context of any minoritized identities you hold. In this case, we invite you to see the comfort of family, friends, and community whom you trust. Whatever multiple identities you hold, we invite you to embody the growth mindset as you read the rest of this chapter.

Historical and Contemporary Contexts

A good place to begin your fine-tuning journey, even if you feel like you have been on it for a while, is to seek out and understand the historical and contemporary contexts that impact people whose identities are minoritized. Step outside of your lens and what you have been taught about this from a dominant perspective. Educate yourself about the pain and suffering that people with minoritized identities have experienced historically and currently. However, do not ask them to educate you. Instead, educate yourself, read memoirs and other writings by people who live with minoritized identities. You may wonder, why not go to the source? For example, why not ask a transgender person to help you learn about their oppressive experiences? The answer is that is it not their job to educate you, that living through the experience is enough without being asked to educate someone who is not transgender. In contrast, people with minoritized identities who write memoirs, blogs, and other readings or documentaries about their lives do that intentionally.

Recognize the trauma that people with minoritized identities hold from legacies of oppression and contemporary manifestations of those legacies. Consider what one of your privileged identities may represent to someone who has lived with the oppression wrought by the power of that unearned privilege. For example, writing from the perspective of Nicole, the second author of this book, I am a white person; this means that I need to read and educate myself about the historical and contemporary oppressive practices toward people of color. I need to take in what my whiteness can represent to people of color. I need to extract what I have done and continue to do to unlearn the racist legacies I have been taught; however, no one can see this work and there may not be any reason a person of color would trust the heart work I've done to unlearn the racism I've been taught. Instead, I need to have humility that there are good historical and contemporary reasons why a person of color may not trust me as a white person. This does not mean that trust cannot be built, that I cannot earn trust, but if it occurs, it happens over time.

One way to move forward on this journey is to use yourself to learn by tapping into any minoritized identities you hold. For example, in addition to my white privilege, I also live with three minoritized identities: as a woman, a lesbian, and an older adult. I build my awareness for what my whiteness can represent to people of color, from my experience of what people who are male presenting, people who are heterosexual, and people who are younger represent to me in terms of the oppressions I experience. To take this even further, as a lesbian and member of the queer community, I am alert to the hatred that many people of faith perpetrate toward those of us in the LGBTQ+ community. This does not mean that I automatically mistrust people who represent these groups. I would be in a sad state if I walked around all the time full of mistrust for so many people and the world. However, what unknown people from those groups represent to me may vary, depending on what else has happened in the past months or what is happening today to activate an experience of oppression due to one of my minoritized identities. The fact that people from these groups with privileged identities may, for me, at first glance not be trustworthy, might feel completely unfair to the kind-hearted man who is doing his work to unlearn misogyny and sexism, or the heterosexual person who, unbeknownst to me, is a staunch ally in the fight for queer rights, or the younger person who has been working to unlearn ageism, or the person of faith who works to help other people of faith unlearn their homophobia. I cannot see that work. The only way I can know it is to build trust, slowly over time, with people as I get to know them.

In summary, educating ourselves is the best way to learn about what any of our privileged identities might represent to someone with a minoritized identity. We invite you to seek out readings and documentaries authored by people who live with minoritized identities and to seek out as many of these sources as possible, because no minoritized identity is a monolith. That is, there is wide diversity of life and experiences within every identity group; no one person can speak for an entire group.

Avoiding Oppressive Curiosities

Oppressive curiosities are questions or statements that pop up in our minds, that may seem harmless and as showing an interest in someone, but that can feel like an insult or invasion of privacy to the person on the receiving end of it. For example, it is common for people who see someone who looks different from them to ask, "Where are you from?" This seems like an innocent thing to be curious about. However, it may not feel like that to the person who is asked the question. Dr. Derald Wing Sue, a scholar and professor of psychology and education, describes his experience of such questions from his position, as an Asian American man. He shares how people will not believe he was born in the United States and keep questioning him, saying things like, "No, really, where are you from?" which sends the message that he is a foreigner in his own land (Sue, 2010). Other examples of oppressive curiosities include asking a gay couple who plays the man and who plays the woman, or asking a person who comes out to you as transgender about their anatomy, or asking someone who uses a wheelchair how they got that way.

We raise this issue of oppressive curiosities because they are typically done from an unconscious and innocent place, but their impact is real. If you want to build trust and work with clients across multiple identities, you need to become aware of how these kinds of questions are experienced. You need to build your self-awareness so that you hear the oppressively curious question in your head before it leaves your mouth. We know that no one reading this book wants to intentionally harm someone in this way. We know, from our own experiences of making mistakes, that the only way to avoid harming someone with oppressively curious questions and comments is to make them visible, to bring them into your conscious awareness. As you will see, this requires work, humility, and commitment. However, we know you will do the work because you want to bring the best of yourself to the clients you serve and the other people in your life.

Oppressive curiosities, accidental ways that we can harm clients with minoritized identities, are more commonly called microaggressions, although there is nothing micro about them (Sue et al., 2019). "Microaggressions are brief, everyday exchanges that send denigrating messages to certain individuals because of their group membership ([e.g.] people of color, women, or LGBTQ+)" (Sue, 2010, p. 24). Sue (2010) goes on to explain that they "often occur outside the level of conscious awareness of well-intentioned perpetrators" (Sue, 2010, p. 40). He (Sue, 2010) states that this is partly what makes them so hideous, because unlike outright and clear oppressive statements about a minoritized group, these kinds of comments occur below our awareness and therefore are much harder to change and unlearn. It is tough to see them because they "are reflections of worldviews that are filled with ethnocentric values, biases, assumptions, and stereotypes that have been strongly culturally inculcated into our beliefs, attitudes, and behaviors" (Sue, 2010, p. 41). Another way to think about this is that these beliefs, attitudes, and behaviors, as Beverly Tatum (1997) states, are like the smog in the air we breathe. Describing cultural racism, she states that it is "like smog in the air. Sometimes it is so thick it is visible, other times it is less apparent, but always day in and day out, we are breathing it in" (Tatum, 1997, p. 6). We can extend this concept of the smog to include all the harmful ideas we have been taught about people with minoritized identities. Day in and day out, we breathe the ideas in, yet we are not even aware of them. The only way to unlearn them and to stop saying them is to build our awareness of them, to make the invisible become visible, to see the smog for what it is, and this requires lifelong learning.

There is an old saying: sticks and stones may break my bones, but names will never hurt me. However, we know this is not true. There is evidence that microaggressions have real impacts on health and wellness of people with minoritized identities (e.g., see Lu et al., 2019; Sawyer et al., 2012; Sue, 2010; Sue, 2019). It is imperative that practitioners take the journey we suggest here to respectfully serve clients across multiple identities.

We close this chapter acknowledging that there are many resources to help you learn about and unlearn the attitudes, beliefs, and behaviors that bubble up inside and spill out in ways that harm people with minoritized identities. Covering these and their complexity is beyond the scope of this book. However, we strongly encourage you to seek out the sources we mention in this chapter and to stay on the lifelong journey of unlearning microaggressions so you can move away from asking questions and making comments that become oppressive curiosities. We suggest a few other sources here that cover topics that are not easily found:

Social Justice Phrase Guide: https://advancementproject.org/resources/the-social-justice-phrase-guide/

Instead of these Ableist Words: https://www.huffpost.com/entry/disability-language-work_l_5f85d522c5b681f7da1c3839

Thirty Everyday Phrases That Perpetuate the Oppression of Indigenous Peoples: https://radicalcopyeditor.com/2020/10/12/thirty-everyday-phrases-that-perpetuate-the-oppression-of-indigenous-peoples/.

Next Chapter

In the next chapter, Chapter 6, we will discuss the risks associated with Experiential Therapy and how to decrease those risks.

Chapter 6
Risk Management

Risk management is the probably the greatest additional consideration when you are integrating Experiential Therapy into your practice. There are few physical risks that a client could experience sitting in a chair in your office. However, moving your furniture to the side so that you and your client(s) can participate in an Experiential Therapy activity or going outside can create an environment where there are more risks. These risks are both physical (falling, tripping, bug bites, etc.) and emotional (being more fully seen, moving in front of others, being in the moment, and feeling like others may be judging them).

Risk-Management Issues to Consider Before Beginning an Experiential Therapy Program

Before you begin an Experiential Therapy program at your organization, make sure you understand your organization's policy on risk and risk assessment. What does the organization see as a risk? What insurance riders does your organization carry? Are there particular policies that pertain to you as an employee or to your clients? Are there policies and procedures that need to be followed that would supersede the ability to do Experiential Therapy? Is the executive director (ED) or clinical director (CD) or principal amenable to your doing Experiential Therapy?

When introducing Experiential Therapy in a new setting that has not previously had an Experiential Therapy program, I usually give a short presentation that includes defining Experiential Therapy, the challenge by choice philosophy, and clinical segues. Then I lead Experiential Therapy activities with staff, and ED, CD, or principals. This allows folks who are in positions of authority to experience the benefits that clients will receive and to become proponents of the modality. Additionally, play is fun for everyone! In some venues, where Experiential Therapy is routinely done, an Experiential Therapy activity is included in monthly staff meetings. This is a bit of a divergence from the topic of risk, but the underscored point is that the more

Understanding and Effectively Utilizing Experiential Therapy. Julie Anne Laser and Nicole Nicotera,
Oxford University Press. © Oxford University Press (2025). DOI: 10.1093/9780197757581.003.0006

that members of the decision-making team are aware and supportive of your Experiential Therapy program, the better it is to do Experiential Therapy in your venue and the more effective you will be.

Risk Management Nuts and Bolts

There are a number of questions you need to ask your human resources team at your organization. First, what sort of insurance does your organization have for you? If you hurt yourself, are you covered? If clients hurt themselves at the office or on the grounds, are they covered by the organization or their own policy? If you hurt yourself outside the office, are you covered? If the client hurts themselves on a trail, are you in danger of being sued? Is there any additional insurance that you should you carry? Is this insurance your responsibility to carry or the organization's responsibility?

You may never need to leave the confines of your office or your organization's yard, but if you were going to hike with clients, what is your work's policy about driving clients? Many organizations are often underinsured when it comes to driving clients. It would be our recommendation that you do not put clients in your car, ever. It would be better to meet the clients at the trailhead where you are going to begin the hike. If the organization has vehicles, then that is a very different situation; you will probably need to get a special license for using those vehicles, and the organization should have a special insurance policy for you to drive.

For your own preparation, it would be prudent to take a course in Wilderness First Aid (WFA) and become certified. WFA classes are offered in many community centers and at many outdoor merchandise stores. They are weekend-long classes that cover basic first aid and the additional issues of exposure to the elements, altitude, wildlife encounters, and first aid considerations when you may be off the grid without telephone service. You will need to refresh your knowledge and skills every 2–3 years to maintain your certification.

It is always necessary to have a first aid kit with you, even if you are just on the premises. It is recommended that you let your clients know that you have a first aid kit as well. We have found this has a secondary benefit in that it also seems to allay fears for anxious clients that safety always comes first, and third, that you always have their back.

Even if you are just going outside the building or going to the park across the street from your office, let someone know from your organization where you are going and when you should be back. You may want to institute a check-out, check-in policy that keeps tabs of where clinicians are during the workday using a simple sign-out, time, location, and expected return time. This is a good safety practice.

Depending on the size of the clinical group and/or the composition of the group, you may need a co-leader. There are no stipulated rules of ratio of clients to therapist, but generally we have found a 1:5 ratio works well when going outside of the office grounds. So if you have a group of 10, you and another clinician will be most effective in co-leading the group in nature.

Risk Management Checklist for Every Client

We have found that a risk management checklist is an effective deterrent to risk for every client. Even if they are members of a family or a couple, every individual needs to fill out their own forms. This does not mean that you will be able to reduce all risks, but it ensures that if there is an issue you will be prepared to act quickly and with the needed information at hand. There should always be three parts to the checklist for every client:

1. **Consent form**: All participants need to fill out a form that they are consenting to be involved in Experiential Therapy activities. The language in our consent form includes the following: "This program can involve strenuous physical activity and may place you/your child in physically, emotionally, and mentally stressful situations. It is important that all participants be in generally good physical condition. Due to the level of physical exertion involved, anyone with health concerns should not participate. Consult with your physician before participating in any physical program." This is not stated to scare clients but to make them aware that there are inherent risks of doing Experiential Therapy. This form should include their full name, today's date, address, cell phone, email, birthdate, and who should be contacted in the case of an emergency and their phone numbers. If they are a minor, their parents will also need to sign the consent form. If they are a minor, they should sign as well, so that they understand that they are giving their permission, which reinforces the challenge by choice philosophy.

2. **Medical form**: Additionally, all participants need to fill out a confidential medical form that includes current and past illnesses both physical and mental, surgeries, chronic medical issues, medications prescribed, allergies (including severity of allergy and intervention needed for allergy), and doctors' names and phone numbers.

3. Copy of their **insurance card**, which is attached to their medical form.

We place these three forms with the other group members' forms in a sealed envelope and carry them in our pack with the first aid kit to all group sessions. This ensures that we always have their emergency contacts, medical information, and insurance card with us if we need it. It is important that clients understand that the information is confidential and is not read by the clinician, other than in the case of an emergency.

Additionally, we have created protocols for each type of Experiential Therapy activity to give as a handout to clients. In the addendum to this chapter, we have shared the general protocol. In Chapter 8, you will find a variety of specific Experiential Therapy in nature protocols. We find that giving them a paper to take home with them or sending it digitally helps the client prepare for the Experiential Therapy session.

Prior to Beginning Experiential Therapy With a New Client

Prior to beginning Experiential Therapy with a new client, you should always conduct an initial intake and assessment with the client. This is usually standard practice in most mental health organizations. This way you know what they want to work on, what issues brought them to therapy, and what motivated them to come to therapy at this time. Additionally, it should ask whether it was their idea or someone else's idea to begin therapy. It should also include any health issues, developmental history, sleep issues, or mobility issues that would preclude them from Experiential Therapy. Are they healthy enough for Experiential Therapy? If unsure, make sure they see a doctor first.

Additionally, you need to really listen to the client. Is the client saying anything that makes you nervous or uncomfortable? Listen to your gut!!!!! If anything they are saying makes you second guess the benefits of leaving the confines of the office, stay in the office doing traditional talk therapy. Some clients should only be seen in the confines of the clinical office due to their being a danger to others or themselves when in a less restricted setting.

Finally, are you personally healthy enough to do Experiential Therapy? Do you have health issues that may preclude your being able to fully engage with clients while being active? Have you seen a doctor recently? Are there medications that you need to carry when going into the outdoors?

If all these issues seem copacetic, then you should explain to the client what Experiential Therapy is, the challenge by choice philosophy, and what clinical segues are, to see if this would be something they would be interested in doing. It is at this point, if they are interested, we would have them fill out the consent form, medical form, and make a copy of their insurance form and give them a specific Experiential Therapy protocol (see Addendum).

Once you are known as an Experiential Therapist in your community, much of this information will have already been conveyed to them prior to coming to work with you, but you should always review the concepts of Experiential Therapy with them to make sure they have understood correctly and to see if they have questions. Additionally, whether they have been to therapy before or not, it is always important to discuss confidentiality, what it is, when you have to break it, and how to maintain confidentiality in the outdoors.

Introducing Current Clients to Experiential Therapy

With current talk therapy clients, you will also need to explain what Experiential Therapy is and the benefits for them, and to fill out the checklist paperwork and give them a specific protocol. We have found that most clients will be cautiously eager to try Experiential Therapy, once they realize it is not "scary." Most will prefer it because it is more "fun" than talk therapy. Remind yourself to go slowly at the pace of the client; remember it is always challenge by choice! But usually, they will enjoy it and find it valuable to their own well-being. As always, you need to uphold the learning zone (window of tolerance) to find activities that are at the right level for them and assess the capacity of each client to manage their own learning zone.

Foreseeable Risks Versus Unforeseeable Risks

When leaving the confines of the office, we need to plan for both the expected and the unknown. First, wherever you go with your client—the community room, gym, backyard of your office, park, or trail—make sure you are personally very familiar with the location. Additionally, you should know in general the number of people who will be in the vicinity of that location at the time you will be there with your client(s). You should be well acquainted with where the bathrooms are, where they can fill up their water bottle, where they can sit down, where they can be in the shade, or where you can run for cover if inclement weather happens. Second, you can never fully eliminate all risk, but the more that you have thought through a good working plan and contingencies to that plan, the better the Experiential Therapy session will be. The importance of careful preparation cannot be overstated.

Thoughtful planning should always include gathering as much relevant information as possible about the client(s), as well as the use of good judgment. Knowledge of the client(s) and a rapport with the client(s) prior to the Experiential Therapy are helpful, though not always possible. There are some particular considerations that make the Experiential Therapy session more successful.

People Outside of Group

As an Experiential Therapist, you need to be vigilant of who may be in the vicinity when you are outside with your client or client group. Make sure that clients are far enough from other nature goers that they are not overheard and, for some, not viewed by others when they are involved in Experiential Therapy activities. Choose areas where you can maintain a good distance from others. Additionally, outside people may be intrigued by the group's activities. Make sure you have a rehearsed response that is both firm and matter of fact that the group is not interested in new members.

Weather

Check and double-check the weather forecast. Make sure you have alternative plans and locations if the weather changes. Make sure that those plans are conveyed to your clients in advance. One year, I was planning to take a group to a challenge course on May 24th and we had 20 inches of snow that morning! We needed to quickly pivot to contact all group members with the information on the new inside venue and to have other activities prepared for them. Also, lightning, hail, and flash floods can happen quickly. Make sure you know your terrain and where you can go for shelter.

What to Bring

Being active means that active clothing and shoes are needed. Each client needs to wear, depending on time of year and weather, a T-shirt, shorts/pants, an insulated jacket (if cooler), sunglasses, sunscreen, socks, closed-toed footwear, and to bring a water bottle, and snacks as needed. This list is provided and discussed with all clients in the protocol prior to the first Experiential Therapy session. If they come ill prepared, we will have to change the activity, or they will have to be an observer and not participant.

Additionally, it is firmly stated that animals, though we love them, often act as a deflection from the Experiential Therapy and should not be brought to sessions. No drugs, alcohol, tobacco, vaping, or weapons are allowed during sessions as well, and this should be overtly stated to avoid confusion. Many of my clients with a military background are often "packing heat," so I address the issue straight on that their weapons, including guns and knives, need to be locked in their car when we are having sessions.

Critters

In Colorado we have bears, mountain lions, bobcats, moose, elk, deer, mountain goats, bighorn sheep, bison, and a variety of snakes, including venomous rattlesnakes. Most of the time, wild animals stay away from humans, but it is not uncommon to see animals from the aforementioned list. We always carry bear spray with us when we a going on nature hikes as a deterrent. But it should only be used as a last resort when the animal is advancing. Most of the time, animals can be better avoided.

Additionally, we have a lot of the small animals—ticks, bees, chiggers, and mosquitoes—that can also be troublesome. You should bring bug spray if going into areas where there are more pests, and clients should wear long sleeves and pants. Additionally, clients should be reminded to check for bites when they return home, and if they have a tick bite they should go to the doctor.

We try to promote Leave No Trace (LNT) principles with our clients to increase their awareness and safety. There are 7 LNT principles (2021): (1) plan ahead and prepare; (2) travel and camp on durable surfaces; (3) dispose of waste properly; (4) leave what you find; (5) minimize your impact; (6) respect wildlife; (7) be considerate of others. These principles help clients know what is expected of them when they are outside, even if it is just the backyard or park. It also helps them understand that they should stay clear of all wildlife and not try to get the "selfie" with the moose!

Injury/Illness

If clients are ill or injured, the planned Experiential Therapy activity may not appropriate. We always have a 24-hour-in-advance cancellation rule: if clients are injured or ill, they should call us 24 hours prior to our session so we can plan a different activity, or they need to reschedule when they are feeling better.

Unexpected Situations

Sometimes you will have a well thought-out plan but an unexpected situation occurs that changes everything, and you have to scrap what you had planned and do something totally different that reflects the current reality or situation. I will give you an example. I was meeting a group of clients to do a late afternoon hike in the mountains. I had arrived about 15 minutes ahead of them. (I always make sure I am in advance of the group so that I can see if there are any changes in the venue from the prior time I was there.) Anyway, when I arrived at the trailhead there were two police officers, and the trailhead was taped off. I inquired why it was closed and the officers said that just a little way down the trail someone had just died by suicide, and they had to wait for the coroner and forensic team to come since it had just happened. I rapidly left the trailhead and waited on the road near the trailhead for my group to arrive. There was no way of contacting them because there was no cell phone coverage. When they arrived, I explained what had happened. We found a picnic bench a little way from the road and talked about ending one's life, the people they had known who had made that choice, and how that had impacted them. It was an intense, sad, and difficult conversation. However, the experience had allowed for a conversation that probably never would have happened that day, if we had not had this experience. It also really moved the group to greater unity, understanding, and appreciation of each other. So sometimes you may have a plan, but there is a different activity that is more important to do instead.

Natural Disasters

As we experience global warming, we have also experienced more forest fires. In Colorado, with increasingly hot and dry summers, it is not uncommon that fires happen. On one occasion, I was meeting a group to hike and as I was arriving at the trailhead, I saw in the distance smoke in the valley. This was where we were planning to hike toward. Once again, there was no cell phone coverage, which meant I needed to wait at the trailhead until the group arrived, and then when they arrived they followed me to a different venue a safe distance from the initial location. Thus, you may be planning to be in a particular venue, but sometimes you need to have other venues that you know well and can use instead, if the need arises.

Activations or Triggers (Known or Unknown)

In the world we live in, where gun violence frequently occurs, it has been suggested that the word "trigger" is often a trigger for individuals who have been witness to, have been involved in, or have known someone who has been hurt or killed by gun violence. Thus, we try to use the verb "activate" or the noun "activation" to describe the feeling of being upset or frightened because they instantly remember something bad in their past, instead of the word "trigger." Sometimes, issues that have been long dormant are activated when your client is in an unfamiliar and somewhat stressful situation. These can be times of new self-awareness, profound growth, and healing. They can also be times of paralyzing fear and sadness, and opportunities for seeing the past event in a new light. Here are two examples:

The first example of self-awareness is that we had just finished an Experiential Therapy activity which will be highlighted in Chapter 11, Ask for Help. The client had come to understand that the way he behaved in the Experiential Therapy activity was exactly how he behaves in his real life, though he expects different outcomes in his real life than what he did in the activity. It was as if he was finally able to see who he was when he interacted with others, rather than just expecting people to behave differently because he wanted them to act differently. He just sat and cried. It was a profound awakening for himself. He realized that so much of what he was doing was pushing people away from him. He realized that friends and family were reacting to him in exactly the way he did not want them to react, but his words and actions were causing that response. It was an "AHA!" moment that he had long kept himself from seeing. This was the turning point in his therapy and an insight into how he could better connect with the important people in his life.

The second example was when I was hiking with a client who was a refugee. As a child, she had had to flee her home in the night and stay several days in hiding in the mountains with her family until they could find safe passage and leave their war-torn country. She dropped to the ground and made herself into a small ball and held her legs and cried. For a moment, I was unsure what had happened to her, and wondered if she was having an acute medical issue. She began to cry and explained that the boulders we were near looked so much like the area around her home where she had hidden with her family. In that moment, she was transported to that time and place. She was re-experiencing the terror, helplessness, and fear of that time in her life.

Once she was able to regain composure, she spoke of her experiences in hiding, the harrowing passage to safety, the loss of her homeland, and the loss of the life she knew. It was an important insight into what had happened, as well as an insight into the very scared little girl that was still having trouble coping, even though the woman she had become was strong and resilient. While it was extremely difficult, it was also a deeply healing experience for her to come to terms with the disparate realities of her past and present. It was also a turning point in her therapy. She could understand what had happened to her as a child in a new and different way, using her adult and not child brain to understand the events. The experience, though difficult, helped to make her more whole and more integrated.

In both these examples, what the client experienced gave them new insights and new ways of understanding themselves and the world around them. The event was a catalyst for growth. Likewise, in both these experiences, it was extremely important to have a trained clinician with them and not merely a wilderness guide or hiking buddy. The very real feelings of being activated needed a trained clinical professional who knows the physical and emotional signs that point to the client's activation and who has the ability to calm, stabilize, and make sense of the experience with the client.

What Is Negligence in Experiential Therapy?

We want to create a plan that minimizes risk as much as possible, while realizing that we can never fully eliminate risk. However, the absence of a well thought-out plan could cause emotional and physical danger for our clients and ourselves. It could also put us in danger of criminal litigation for being neglectful. Noted recreation and adventure sports law attorney, Tracey Knutson states:

> Negligence under the law is generally defined as the failure to use ordinary care; that is, failing to do what a person of ordinary prudence would have done under the same or similar circumstances. Essentially, we are looking to determine whether an operator, educator, clinician, or land administrator could or should have recognized an unreasonable risk and then did nothing to warn the participant or to reduce or eliminate the unreasonable risk. To examine negligence in behavior or conduct, look for 2 things: was the risk foreseeable and was the risk unreasonable. (www.traceyknutson.com)

Thus, planning to reduce and avoid risk as much as possible and not taking unnecessary risks keep us from being neglectful. Remember that safety is always our biggest concern.

Emotional Safety in a New Group

We have discussed the importance of reducing risk regarding the client's physical safety. We now turn our attention into how we can best increase emotional safety in a new group.

Build Rapport

How do you simultaneously build connection to new group members and make sure you are in control of the group's safety? We first need to be clear what our role is as a clinician and facilitator. We need to provide safety and security for the group members to express themselves and grow, but also warmth and comfortability to know that our group is a safe place.

Create a Group Contract

One way we can help build rapport is through a group contract. The group contract at its essence articulates what is acceptable and what is not, as a group member. We have found that the group contract works best if we co-create the group contract in the first session of the group. We ask the group members to be specific; for example: hands are for helping not hurting, no put-downs, no name calling, no bullying, no mimicking, no demeaning, no mocking, no discussion of sexual predilections, no discussion of substance use (unless a substance abuse group), no discussion of illegal activities, what language is okay to use in group, and what language is not okay to use. We write the tenets of the contract down on a piece of paper so that we can refer to it in future group sessions when necessary. Once created, the contract is agreed upon by all group members. It is the first activity that begins to create an identity and shared purpose of the group.

Confidentiality Within the Group

Additionally, during the first session, there needs to be a discussion of confidentiality. We explain what confidentiality is and the importance of supporting all group members to feel they are in a safe place, where group members can say what they truly feel. However, it is also a reality that humans sometimes like to gossip about unusual or troubling issues they have heard with their own people. Even though we ask for confidentiality for what we discuss in group, there is no "confidentiality police." Thus, we let group members know that they can talk to us personally before or after the session as needed if they do not feel comfortable sharing with the entire group. As time goes on and greater trust is felt between group members, greater sharing happens in the group and much less before- or after-group individual sharing.

A Commitment to Address and Uphold Emotional Safety

In the first group sessions, you will feel that you are the hub of the group and each group member is one of the spokes of the wheel, but as the group develops, the group members create relationships to each other and you do not need to be such an influential leader, but can have the group work collectively. We particularly like the Tuckman and Jensen (1977) stages of the group to understand group development. Though the stages do not universally proceed in the manner they suggest all of the time, having the expectancy that generally most groups will proceed through these stages is very useful. These stages are: forming, storming, norming, performing, and adjourning.

Forming

In the forming stage, the group is tasked with identifying who is who, what the group rules are, and how group members fit in. The clinician needs to ensure safety and acceptance of all group members and give guidance. Experiential Therapy activities are very low risk, such as activities that help group members remember each other's names and general information about each other.

Storming

In the second stage of group development, there is often, but not always, conflict and competition. The group members begin to know each other better and behaviors and personalities sometimes grate upon each other. The therapist needs to model tolerance and to coach group members to move through this stage. This can mean that the clinician needs to gently squash issues that will decrease group effectiveness, such as a group member who tries to commandeer the group or the Experiential Therapy activity. Sometimes, some group struggles are good and productive for creating future group cohesion, in that they have together overcome a barrier of understanding.

Conflict is not always a bad thing, and sometimes having had to work through an issue makes the group stronger and more resilient. However, if the conflict turns into disrespect of group members, then the group has to return to the group contract, and civility needs to be restored in the group by the therapist.

Norming

In the third stage, some of the difficulties of the storming stage are being further worked out. There is increased cohesion, sharing, and trust building within the group. The Experiential Therapy activities can support group members in bringing their authentic self to sessions and allow for greater vulnerability. The clinician models support of the group members and begins to move from being the focus of the group discussion to watching and supporting the group members interact with each other.

Performing

In the fourth stage, the group has become integrated. There are feelings of unity within the group. A shared group identity emerges, and there is interdependence between group members. Group members are comfortable allowing themselves to be fully seen, heard, and acknowledged. The therapist is no longer the hub of the group and can delegate responsibilities to other group members. The group has the skills, trust, and knowledge of each other to be fully present as themselves in the Experiential Therapy activities.

Adjourning

The group is moving to the completion of the group. Group members are acknowledging the skills and competencies that increased while they were a group member and their own growth as a human. The therapist facilitates each group member to recognize each other group member's contribution to the group. The clinician supports the closure of the group and perhaps creates a graduation from the group in the form of a certificate or a memento or closing activity (see Chapters 10 and 11). Rituals of graduation can often be effective in closing the group to help group members acknowledge their own and everyone else's contribution, growth, and successful completion of the group. Framing it as a successful completion is extremely important for many group members who have not been successful in completing other tasks or who have not experienced the joy of graduation.

These stages are helpful expectancies of group development. However, not all groups will move through all of these stages because of time constraints of the group or personalities within the group. But when a group does move through the stages, as a therapist it is a beautiful thing to behold, because you have given the clients a supportive network that can support them after the group officially terminates. In some instances, I have heard that the friendships that the group created were still functioning years after the group ended.

Characteristic of the Therapist to Support Emotional Safety in Experiential Therapy

Positive Attitude

In the fable of the sun and the wind, the sun and the wind make a bet of who can get the individual down on earth to remove their coat. The wind goes first and blows hard and strong and the only thing the individual does is to hold more forcefully on to their coat. But then the sun comes out and shines bright and warm, and the individual under their own volition takes off their coat themselves. Thus, be the sun! There may be days you may not feel like being the sun, but the group or the individual did not come to hear your own personal problems or issues. They came to work on themselves. A benefit of this is that you also may feel better yourself by acting like the sun.

A Willingness to Allow the Group to Struggle a Bit

As stated already, a little struggling is good for the group's development and cohesion. Coming to the group's aid too quickly stifles their development. Allow for times of quiet reflection and pregnant pauses. Sometimes silence allows the group to process and to think more clearly. Successful completion of Experiential Therapy activities does not happen right away. Allow the group to try, fail, and try something new and better than the last attempt. This helps them feel that they have really accomplished the task and gives them a sense of pride and makes the group more cohesive.

Cultural Sensitivity

The better that you understand the culture where your clients come from, the better that you can support their growth. Make sure you consider gender, age, language, sexual identity, sexual expression, race, ethnicity, country of origin, religious tenets, and trauma history when putting group members together in pairs or smaller groups. Some group members will not like to be in close proximity to others. Others will not want anyone to touch them during a group activity or maintain eye contact for too long. The more that you understand who they are and their needs as group members, the better you can support their having a positive experience.

Flexibility and a Willingness to Try New Things

The best laid plans are not always the ones that you will use on a given day, as already stated. The more that you can be responsive to the needs of the group and get a pulse of the group, the better the session will be. I often will bring three or four Experiential Therapy activities when I am only planning to do two activities during the session. This allows me to choose between activities that better align to the energy level and the emotions of the group.

Style That Is Authentic to Yourself

Do not perform as the "therapist"; be you. If they believe you to be authentic, they will bring their authentic selves, too! If they see you for you, they will be more open to be seen as themselves. This means that a lot more work can be done in sessions.

These characteristics help the Experiential Therapist make every session an opportunity for growth and self-discovery. They will also help you truly enjoy your work.

Next Chapter

In the next chapter, we will discuss how we structure Experiential Therapy activities over time.

Addendum

Experiential Therapy General Protocol

Expected Time

Purpose/Objective

To use experiential activities as a tool for doing experiential therapy. This is an opportunity to participate in experiential therapy activities with family/partner/group and clinician. The activities are often a catalyst to discuss issues impacting their lives.

Certifications and Qualifications of Therapist(s)

Put your name and qualifications here

Age, Gender, Physical Ability, and Cultural Considerations

Need parental consent if under 18
    Need to be healthy to be involved in this activity; get medical approval prior to being involved

Equipment/Materials Needed

- Clothing: comfortable clothing
- Closed-toed shoes (athletic shoes or hiking boots)
- Sunglasses (if outside)
- Water in water bottle
- Snacks as needed
- Suntan lotion
- Bug spray

Disclaimer: If the client does NOT wear appropriate attire and have good working equipment per the therapist's estimation, she/he/they will not be able to participate in the activity.

Risk Assessment

Prerequisites

Need to be healthy to participate in this activity; get doctor's approval.

Risks You May Be Exposed to

- Allergies (bring meds or inhaler if necessary)
- Injury (Therapist will have first aid kit; however, if there is a fall, medical care may be needed)
- Unpredictability of nature—weather, wildlife, terrain, sunburn

How to Best Prepare Yourself for This Activity

What Not to Bring:

- No animals
- No drugs/alcohol
- No weapons
- No tobacco (no nicotine products, including vaping)

Check weather before session

If you have any questions, feel free to contact the therapist before the activity.

Be aware of road conditions on your way to the activity, as well.

All suitability for activities will be evaluated upon intake with the therapist. If you have any questions or concerns, please communicate these with your therapist any time before, during, or after the activity.

Chapter 7
Structuring Experiential Therapy Interventions

We have created a standardized template for all Experiential Therapy Activities. We use a 10-step outline for this template. This helps us create common terminology and create greater interrater reliability (ensuring that Experiential Therapists are doing the same Experiential Therapy activity the same way). The 10 steps are: (1) name of activity; (2) time duration; (3) purpose/objective; (4) age/gender/cultural considerations; (5) equipment/materials needed; (6) risk assessment; (7) framing questions; (8) directions for activity; (9) clinical segues and questions; (10) for whom would this activity be appropriate, and for whom would it not be appropriate?

Name of Activity

What is the activity called? The name is important because the clients can refer to the name of the activity in future sessions to discuss the activity and how they showed up in the activity. A humorous name adds a playful touch and may help with buy-in. The name also may help the client begin to understand what the Experiential Therapy activity will be.

Time Duration

How long will it take to successfully complete the Experiential Therapy activity? This is always a guesstimate, and individuals and groups could take more or less time than suggested. But it gives a good estimation of whether there is enough time in the session to complete the activity.

Purpose/Objective

What should the clients gain by doing the activity? What is the end goal?

Understanding and Effectively Utilizing Experiential Therapy. Julie Anne Laser and Nicole Nicotera,
Oxford University Press. © Oxford University Press (2025). DOI: 10.1093/9780197757581.003.0007

Age/Gender/Cultural Considerations

Do participants need to be a certain age to intellectually understand the activity? Is there physical contact (e.g., holding hands or putting hands on shoulders) that may be inappropriate for some individuals to do because of age, gender, or cultural or religious mores?

Equipment/Materials Needed

What materials or equipment are needed to complete the activity? Sometimes no materials or equipment are needed other than sufficient space for the clients to be able to move. Other times particular equipment or props are needed to make the Experiential Therapy activity successful. Can you purchase these materials one time and reuse them? Or do you need to purchase new materials every time you do the particular Experiential Therapy activity?

Sometimes Experiential Therapy activities require renting equipment. Always rent from a reputable outdoor equipment vendor to get high-quality well-maintained equipment for outdoor activities. We have found that if you establish a relationship with the outdoor rental organization, they will rent equipment to your group members at a reduced rate. Additionally, there may be charges to visit a particular venue and reservations in advance may need to be made.

Risk Assessment

There should never be more than minimal risk involved in the Experiential Therapy activity. But there are emotional risks in a new group that need to be considered so that the risk of sharing too much when they are not ready, the risk of failure in front of others, the risk of being vulnerable in front of others, the risk of the unknown, and the risk of being seen in a new or different light do not happen until the participants are ready to do so.

Framing Questions

These are the questions that should guide the clients' entrance into the Experiential Therapy activity. What should the clients' mindset be when they begin the Experiential Therapy activity? This is different than the purpose or objective because it is the entrance into the activity, not the outcome of the activity.

Directions for Activity

What are the steps, rules, and instructions for carrying out the Experiential Therapy activity to completion? Sometimes there are a lot of directions. However, sometimes there are purposefully fewer directions so that the individual or group has to generate ideas, try their ideas, and refine their ideas to complete the activity.

Clinical Segues and Questions

Clinical segues are the process in which the Experiential Therapy activity becomes Experiential Therapy. It is transferring the learning from what just happened to what can be taken with them, today, tomorrow, and always. It is making the Experiential Therapy activities connect to the clients' life in and outside of therapy. The questions asked to the clients can help them center and ground the activity. Clinical segues provide clients an opportunity to gain deeper understandings about life and living, whether the Experiential Therapy activity was fun, exciting, frustrating, or difficult. For instance, what did they learn about themselves and group members? Does this resemble how they show up in other spheres of their life?

Clients, through clinical segues, can gain insights into: who they really are, what is important to them, what they can control in their lives, what strengths they actually possess, who in their lives can they count on, what they really want to do in their lives, what makes them happy, what the next steps are to make their goals a reality, who really knows them, who really understands them, what they have been hiding from themselves, what they have been hiding from others and why, what they have been holding on to that they don't need any longer, what they are grieving, why they feel shame, why they feel loss, why they feel abandonment, what makes them anxious, what makes them feel lonely, what makes them feel frustrated. So the Experiential Therapy activity becomes a catalyst for discussing a myriad of topics that have long existed within the client, but are now more accessible to discuss because of the Experiential Therapy activity that they participated in.

For Whom Would This Activity Be Appropriate, and for Whom Would It Not Be Appropriate?

To be honest, not every experiential activity is for everyone. Do clients have physical limitations that cannot be overcome? Are there modifications to the Experiential Therapy activity that need to be made because of a vision impairment, hearing impairment, mobility issues, neurodivergent issues, or maturity issues? Are there members in the group for whom being their authentic selves would be too activating at the present time to do the Experiential Therapy activity? Perhaps the Experiential Therapy activity needs to be introduced later when the group is more solidly connected? Additionally, particular Experiential Therapy activities may activate a person who has experienced a particular life event. The clearer you are about whom the activity would be appropriate for, the more enjoyable and insightful the Experiential Therapy activity will be for the client.

Ratcheting up the Experiential Therapy Activities Over Sessions

Many clinical issues at their root are related to trauma and grief. But these clinical issues may show up in their lives being masked as substance abuse, acting out behavior, violence, illegal activities, depression, anxiety, rudeness, problems with relationships, or lack of interest (apathy). Successive Experiential Therapy activities can help clients take off the mask permanently. When we organize successive Experiential Therapy activities, they help the individual grow and reach a little bit more in each session. This helps clients increase insights over time, decrease effects of trauma, and increase resilience. In groups, it helps them allow themselves to be more fully seen and heard as their authentic selves.

Staying out of the Panic Zone

As stated in Chapters 1 and 3, we need to always be aware of where the client is in the client's therapeutic window (Briere, 2002); in Experiential Therapy, we use the terms *relax zone, learning zone,* and *panic zone* with clients to let us know how they are feeling internally and to get a quick read from clients during the Experiential Therapy activities. But we should also be continually assessing facial and body signs and movements that signal that they are nearing the panic zone or are becoming activated. We need to not only ask them how they are feeling, but also assess for signs of mounting activation. For some clients, they will have a hard time assessing themselves personally because they have spent so much time being activated that they are unable to self-assess well. We have found that if they have the option to wear an athletic watch or heart monitor, they can learn how to better understand what their body feels like when it is stressed and learn what it feels like to reduce their stress. Obviously, not all clients can afford such devices, but they give real feedback to those who can; if there are monies available at your organization, it may be possible to purchase them and lend them to clients during Experiential Therapy activities.

Stages of Trauma Therapy

When we begin to allow for greater vulnerability in the group, we need to make sure we are in alignment with the stages of trauma therapy (Herman, 1992, 2015). They are: (1) building trust with the client(s); (2) creating empathy and understanding; (3) ensuring that therapy is client focused and at client's pace; (4) instilling hope that they will feel better; (5) allowing them to tell their own story; (6) helping them understand that what happened to them does not define who they are; (7) building hope for the future; (8) finding meaning in their story and putting their story into the greater meaning of their life (Herman, 1992, 2015). Following these stages will help them to connect in therapy to you and to others if they are in a group. It also helps you follow their pace and timing of therapy. If you push them in therapy too much when they are not ready, they will not return or will take a hiatus from therapy.

Grief

It has been stated that "all grief does not have trauma, but ALL trauma has grief" (David Kessler, Grief Educator Training, May 10, 2023). To work through grief with clients, there are six needs that must be addressed in therapy (Kessler, 2020). The first need is that the pain of grief must be witnessed. The pain of grief needs to be normalized as part of loss and part of love.

Grief is a natural outcome of having loved. Bottling up grief is not good for the grieving person; it needs to be witnessed by others. Therapy is often the perfect place for that witnessing to occur.

The second need is that the grieving person should try to express their feelings (Kessler, 2020). Often grief stifles the client's vocabulary of feeling anything other than sad, angry, or hurt. Sometimes if they do not have an ample vocabulary regarding feelings, the clinician needs to help the client learn "feeling" words in order to talk about their emotions, which can often be complex or contradictory. All feelings should be discussed without attaching good or bad to the feelings; they simply are.

The third need of grief is to release the burden of guilt (Kessler, 2020). Often the client is stuck in the "would have, could have, should have" scenario of the loss. Guilt gives us a false sense of control (Kessler, 2020), that there was something we could have done, and the outcome would have been different. However, the reality almost always is that in the "what if" or "only if" scenarios, the outcome would be the same, "even if" we were able to do something (Kessler, 2020). The client needs to realize that they did not and do not possess the ability, insight, or omnipresence to have changed the outcome.

The fourth need for clients is to realize that often in grief, old wounds are brought to the surface when the new wounds of grief are felt, and that both need healing (Kessler, 2020). Often long forgotten or deeply hidden injustices, arguments, or memories resurface with the new grief. These old wounds may complicate or undermine the client's ability to grieve. The new grief needs to be witnessed and the old wounds need to be brought into the light to be discussed and understood.

The fifth need is to integrate pain and love together (Kessler, 2020). "A broken heart is also an open heart" (David Kessler, Grief Educator Training, May 10, 2023). The pain of grief is only because we have loved the individual who is no longer in our lives. Pain and love all come from loving the individual.

The sixth need is to not stop at acceptance, but to find meaning in what has happened (Kessler, 2020). Kessler states, "Grief does not get smaller, we have to become bigger" (David Kessler, Grief Educator Training, May 10, 2023). "Once you find your way through the pain, you will find amazing meaning underneath and that meaning transforms us" (David Kessler, Grief Educator Training, May 10, 2023). We need to reframe grief as an opportunity for growth, new learning, and understanding new perspectives of life and living.

Grounding Exercises

When we feel that the client is getting close to being activated, we can employ a variety of grounding activities to help them firmly stay in the learning zone, as discussed in Chapter 3.

1, 2, 3, 4, 5

If you notice the client on the verge of becoming activated: (1) Ask them to sit down (if outside), or to sit down and face a window (if indoors). (2) Ask them to close their eyes, and focus on their breathing. (3) Then ask them to slowly open their eyes; what do they see? (4) What do they hear? (5) What do they smell? This simple activity helps clients break the cycling thoughts, and to turn their senses to something new. Once they learn the activity, they can employ the activity anytime they need.

Stop, Challenge, Choose

This is a quick Cognitive Behavioral Therapy (CBT) activity called Stop, Challenge, Choose (Wilson & Wilson, 2004) to stop rumination, to refocus, to choose an alternative solution, to end circling conversations that are going nowhere. We have found that if you teach this during a session, then the clients can do it on their own whenever they need it. The first step is to **Stop**: The client needs to be encouraged to mentally disconnect from the situation or conversation, to breathe, and to recenter themselves. Then they need to take a moment to observe how their body is doing.

The second step is to **Challenge** what are they thinking. What are they telling themselves? What are they making up and why? What past experience are they connecting the current one to? What are they believing that is causing their current feelings? What are the objective data that support these negative feelings? What are other possible interpretations of the situation?

The third step is to **Choose**. What is their best response? Is it based on objective or factual data? Is the response in their best long-term interest? Then, they should choose it and use it instead.

Dealing With Difficult Feelings: Four Steps

Once again, teach this in session, and then clients can do it anytime they need. (1) Notice the feeling. (2) Name the feeling. (3) Sit with the feeling. (4) Let the feeling go. We have found if you pretend to blow the feeling away, it adds an action to letting the feeling go.

Five-Minute Vacation

This is another activity that helps clients recenter and refresh when they are feeling they may be getting activated. Once again, teach this in session, and then it is theirs to use whenever they need it. Ask the client to sit comfortably with their eyes shut, or at least not looking at anyone. Ask them to think of a place that they love (a beach, a forest, a park bench, grandma's kitchen table, a mountain, their friend's house, their sofa at home, etc.). Have them spend a moment thinking of that lovely place and really visualizing it. Then have them bring in the rest of their senses to their mind's eye. What does it feel like? Is it hot or cold? Is there a breeze? Is it day or night? What noises do you hear? What does it smell like? If you could taste the food there, what would it taste like? Let them reminisce about that place for about five minutes and then ask them to slowly open their eyes again. They should feel renewed and refreshed.

Tapping

Tapping is another alternative to use when the client is feeling activated (The Tapping Solution Foundation, 2024). The client is directed to lightly touch with their fingertips different meridian points of their body. They should lightly tap each meridian point 5–7 times before moving to the next one. The meridian points are: the top of the head, above the eyebrows, under the eye on the cheekbone, under the nose, on the chin bone, on the collarbones, under the arm, and one the side of the hand from the knuckle of the pinky to the wrist (The Tapping Solution Foundation, 2024). At first, you will need to remind them of the meridian points, but once they remember them, they can use them anytime they need them. These should feel calmer and more able to be present again.

Mantras

Having something they can say to themselves when they are feeling activated helps them reduce those feelings. A mantra can be used as a go-to phrase that they say to themselves whenever they need to be soothed. The mantra can be a phrase that they have made up themselves, or it can be borrowed from the many mantras available. Mainly they should either have it with them, in their wallet to read over, or have it memorized so it is there any time they need it. Creating a mantra can be done in session or they can use one that they like. We have found that some particularly good ones are: doubt the doubt; be a buffalo not a cow (buffalo run through the storm to the other side, cows run away from the storm and invariably the storm catches them; David Kessler, Grief Educator Training, May 10, 2023); forgiveness is a gift you give yourself; do the best you can, and when you know better, do better (Maya Angelou); this too shall pass; you are stronger than you think you are; no feeling is final; and touch the pain and then take a break (David Kessler, Grief Educator Training, May 10, 2023). They also may want to write these mantras down and put them on their bathroom mirror or refrigerator as well.

Metaphors in Nature

When outside with clients, nature gives great examples of metaphors that can reduce activation. Metaphors in nature can include: the deep roots of tree that can withstand the harshest winds; the solidity of a rock; the meandering though purposeful movement of a river; the tenacity of a plant growing to the light; the bending and not breaking of the trunk of a tree by the wind; the ability of a small beaver to change the direction of a powerful river; the flight of migratory birds who have both flown a long way and have a long way still to go. All can be used to support clients to feel calmed and to change their current thinking.

You will find that particular clients will prefer different grounding activities. They will sometimes use one for a while and then begin to use another. Some clients will find some grounding techniques silly, and others will love it and use it all the time. This is why it is such a good idea to share with them a wide variety of techniques.

Experiential Therapy Activities

We have included three examples of Experiential Therapy Activities in this chapter. The first is a very low-risk, low-vulnerability activity called All My Neighbors. We often use this as an opening activity for the first session. It helps group members learn each other's names and is a fun activity. The second Experiential Therapy activity is called Beach Ball Emotions. It has a little bit more vulnerability in the activity because clients are talking about an emotion that they have felt. This activity also helps clients increase their "feeling" vocabulary and can be used for that purpose as well. The third is still a little more vulnerable because they need to talk not only about the emotion, but also how they relate to another's sentence about the emotion. Lastly, if you are doing Experiential Therapy in nature, we also want you to see how you ratchet it up over time.

All My Neighbors

Time Duration: 20 minutes

Purpose/Objective: The purpose of the activity is to recognize individual strengths and capabilities and to support individual differences and commonalities in the group. It also helps the group know each other's names.

Age/Gender/Cultural Considerations: None

Equipment/Materials Needed: Enough plastic/paper plates for every participant, minus one

Risk Assessment: Low risk, as long as movement between plates is done safely. There is some risk of self-disclosure.

Framing Questions: What makes us unique? How are we similar to the rest of the group?

Directions for Activity:

1. Arrange plates in a circle, with one less plate than participants.
2. Remind them that we will not be sharing information about ourselves that could possibly get us in trouble (e.g., sexual escapades, substance use, or illegal behavior).
3. Anytime they have had a particular experience, they need to change the plate they were standing on so they are at least 2 places away from it. For instance: "All of my neighbors who like to ski/snowboard move across the circle like a skier or snowboarder" OR "All of my neighbors who have visited Mexico, move across the circle in giant steps" OR "All of my neighbors who have lived in more than four different homes in their lives move across the circle on tip toes," OR "All of my neighbors who like to bake cross the circle while pretending to mix a bowl of batter." Encourage creativity in both finding qualities that are unknown by the other group members and silly ways of crossing the circle, but that also may apply to a variety of group members.
4. You should be the first leader and stand in the middle of the circle, You should say your name, and then have them all respond, "Hello . . . "; then you state, "All of my neighbors who . . . (you must have this attribute too)".

5. Everybody who possesses this attribute needs to cross the circle in the way they are instructed to walk, they must find a plate that is not immediately next to them.
6. You quickly go to a new plate along with everyone else who possesses the quality.
7. The new leader is the person who is left standing without standing on a plate and repeats the process from the middle of the circle: "Hello, my name is. . . . All of my neighbors who. . . ."
8. Play until everyone has the opportunity to be the leader.

Clinical Segues and Questions: Did you learn new information about group members? Are you surprised you are with such an interesting and talented group? Did you realize you have more similarities to other group member than originally thought? When you were the leader, did you find yourself trying to find similar interests to other group members? Did it feel comfortable, or uncomfortable, to let the group know something about yourself when you were the leader?

For Whom Would This Activity Be Appropriate, and for Whom Would It Not Be Appropriate? The activity can be played with all age groups.

Beach Ball Emotions

Time Duration: 10–30 minutes

Purpose/Objective: To identify and remember recent emotions they have had

Age/Gender/Cultural Considerations: Clients must be able to read and to catch a beach ball thrown gently from a short distance.

Equipment/Materials Needed: A beach ball with names of emotions written with permanent marker over the surface of the beach ball. Some emotion words that could be included are: love, pride, happiness, sadness, anger, joy, frustration, loneliness, encouragement, excitement, energy, comfortable, calm, supported, trusted, understood, sympathetic, loss, misunderstood, undervalued, interested, accepted, kind, happy, great, joyous, lucky, delighted, thankful, fortunate, cheerful, playful, optimistic, peaceful, surprised, relaxed, reassured, considerate, passionate, admiration, intrigued, fascinated, hopeful, dynamic, cherished, needed, treasured.

Risk Assessment: There is no physical real risk other than perhaps being hit by the ball. If the emotion is a hard one for them, they may not want to share with the group.

Framing Question: Discuss a time when you felt that emotion recently?

Directions for Activity:

1. Have the group make a circle.
2. One client throws the ball to another client.
3. That client catches the ball.
4. The client who caught the ball notices where their thumbs are on the beach ball and the two "feeling" words that are closest to each thumb.
5. The client who caught the ball explains a time when they felt those emotions. They can share both emotion words that are nearest to both thumbs; or if they do not want to discuss one of the them, they can opt to discuss only one of the emotions; or if they do not like either emotion, they can throw the ball up and recatch the ball, to discuss to different emotions where their thumbs are.
6. The ball is then thrown to another client, and the game continues.
7. The activity is completed when everyone has caught the ball at least once. The activity can be played through a second or third round depending on time and interest.

Clinical Segues and Questions: How was it to state the feelings you had in front of the group? Was it easier to state the more "positive" or more "negative" emotions? Why do you think that was the case? If others had the same emotion, was it easier to hear what others said than to give your response? How did it feel to remember those emotions? Are there emotions you wish your thumb was on? Were there emotions you did not want to discuss? Why?

For Whom Would This Activity Be Appropriate, and for Whom Would It Not Be Appropriate? For those with mobility issues, the ball could be rolled across a table. For neurodivergent clients, they may have some difficulty in stating a time they felt that emotion.

Fear in a Hat; Pride in a Hat (Any Emotion in a Hat)

Time Duration: 15–20 minutes

Purpose/Objective: This activity is meant to take a mindful and caring tone. Facilitator should remind participants to keep in mind the concept of empathy while participating, as expressing fears (or the emotion chosen) may place some in a vulnerable state. This activity's purpose is to allow clients to express current fears (or other emotions) that they have in regard to their life and for others to be able to relate to those fears (or other emotions). It is an opportunity to share feelings about the emotions in a nonjudgmental space.

Age/Gender/Cultural Considerations: Modifiable based on development. Modifications could include Wishes in a Hat, Likes/Dislikes in a Hat, Worries in a Hat, Pride in a Hat.

This activity does not have to be centered on fears, and should be done only if the group is ready and willing to share emotions and feelings.

Equipment/Materials Needed: A hat, writing utensils, and small pieces of paper

Risk Assessment: Minimal physical risk with medium emotional risk, as this activity requires some level of vulnerability

Framing Question: How do we experience vulnerability through sharing our experiences of an emotion, and how do we accept group support through acceptance and empathy?

Directions for Activity:

1. Direct participants to make a circle in a seated position.
2. Pass out pens and paper to clients.
3. Place the hat in the middle of the circle.
4. Ask clients to complete one of these sentences anonymously, the same sentence for everyone:
   a. "I have fear about . . ."
   b. "I am proud of . . ."
   c. "I am sad about . . ."
   d. "I feel lonely about . . ."
   e. "I feel excited about . . ."
5. Tell participants they have three minutes to write down their answers.
6. Remind participants to not write their names on their papers.
7. Once participants finish writing, have them place their paper in the hat.
8. Shuffle the papers.
9. Tell the group that the hat will be passed around in the circle and that each participant will take one piece of paper, reading aloud the sentence.
10. No other participant besides the reader is allowed to comment on the sentence.
11. The reader will reflect on the sentence, and comment how they relate to the feeling and the sentence they just read.
12. Throughout the activity make sure all participants are listening and not commenting.
13. After all the papers have been read aloud, discuss.
14. Do the activity again with a different emotion.

Clinical Segues and Questions: How did it feel to have your sentence read aloud? Did it feel good that someone else could relate to your sentence? Did this activity bring up any other feelings for you? How did you address these feelings as they were coming up? How do you see this activity helping us grow as a group? Do you think this activity has helped foster a sense of support within our group? Do you feel like you know each other better?

For Whom Would This Activity Be Appropriate, and for Whom Would It Not Be Appropriate? This activity is appropriate for youth and adults, not children. If clients are neurodiverse, they may not be able to relate to what is written on the paper. The group needs to not be in the early stages of formation; rapport and trust need to be felt between group members. The feelings may need to be bounded by a particular sphere of their lives, for instance, fears at school, fears for the future, and so on. Since the sentences are anonymous, if someone writes something that is troubling, the author will not be known, so it is important to have insights into group members.

Ratcheting up in Nature

The same progression happens in doing Experiential Therapy in nature. We may begin Experiential Therapy by meeting at a park. We may walk for a bit or spend most of the session on a park bench. From that session we may feel that another bench sit is appropriate for the pace of therapy. Or conversely, we may venture to walk around the park in the next session. From there we may move to a nearby trail.

Next Chapter

In Chapter 8, we will more fully discuss Experiential Therapy in nature.

Chapter 8
Experiential Therapy in the Natural Realm

John Muir (1838–1914), noted naturalist and father of the U.S. national park system, stated, "in every walk with nature one receives far more than they seek" (Klimes & Klimes, 1986, p. 53). As discussed in Chapter 2, there is an inherent, deep connection of human beings to natural spaces. Experiential Therapy in nature uses that long-standing and robust relationship with nature to support growth in the individual and/or group. Bringing clients outside has recently increased in popularity as a clinical practice, and it has even been recently reported by the *New York Times* that "therapists trade their couch for the great outdoors" (Caron, February 5, 2024). Thus, the world is beginning to take notice of the practice and benefits of bringing clients outside.

However, as stated in Chapter 6, moving clients from the office to the outdoors creates a whole host of new considerations. Thus, doing Experiential Therapy in nature necessitates careful consideration of risks and an array of strategies to reduce those risks. It means creating a good plan and flexibility to create alternative plans if needed. Just as a reminder: You must have each client's health information and release information already and bring them with you when you leave the confines of your office. You will need to always carry a first aid kit with you, even if it is just to the backyard. If they have any allergy or asthma issues, you should make sure they have their medications before going outside. If you are meeting the client(s) in another location, you should reiterate with client(s) the location where you will be meeting, the duration of the activity, what to bring, what to do if there are weather issues, and a Plan B if you need to cancel the outdoor activity or change location.

The second part of this chapter shares protocols for a wide variety of outdoor activities: walking, hiking, challenge course, road biking, camping, paddleboarding, and snowshoeing. This will give you a good sense of how to do these or similar activities in any season of the year.

Understanding and Effectively Utilizing Experiential Therapy. Julie Anne Laser and Nicole Nicotera,
Oxford University Press. © Oxford University Press (2025). DOI: 10.1093/9780197757581.003.0008

So, What Do We Do With Clients Outside?

There are many similarities of doing clinical therapy inside to doing therapy outside. In fact, the major issues you will discuss are exactly the same; it is how they are delivered that is different. For instance, if you are working with a client discussing their trauma story, this can easily and effectively be done on a trail, a walk, paddleboarding, biking, or snowshoeing. We have found that in many ways, telling the trauma story is much easier in nature because the client does not feel the need to maintain eye contact with the therapist, since they need to look where they are going. The client can also pause for a moment to take in the natural world around them, collect their thoughts, and continue telling their story. When in the office, those pauses are fraught with more anxiety and tension for the client, and sometimes for the therapist as well. Additionally, on a hike or a walk, or on a paddleboard, a bike ride, or snowshoeing, the pace of conversation is often slowed down to take in the natural world around them, perhaps to breathe in the fresh air, take a sip of water from their water bottle, and to reflect on what they have said and what they want to say. It is always at the speed of the client. Therapy in nature, therefore, seems more natural, less forced, and less awkward.

Beginning the Activity in Nature

Often before we begin an Experiential Therapy activity in nature with a group, we bring a rope that has been tied into a circle. We call this activity "hope, fears, goals." We ask the clients to each hold on to the rope with one hand. We slowly have the rope go through their hands, and when the knot comes to their hand in the first round, they can state a hope for the activity (if they choose, because it is always challenge by choice); when everyone on the circle has had the knot pass through their hands and has completed their hope, the rope moves in the other direction and fears are shared by all who choose to participate; the rope travels in the other direction one more time for the discussion of goals. We have found that this activity sets the stage for the day's intentions and can help keep clients focused and present with what is happening during their time in nature, rather than thinking about what has happened before they arrived or what will be happening later.

Intention words can also be chosen at the beginning of an Experiential Therapy activity in nature to help consider the word throughout the activity for the individual client or group. There are a multitude of words that could be chosen, but some words that we have found to be particularly effective are: gratitude, grace, serenity, peace, growth, rebirth, renewal, resilience, transcendence, development, and the circle of life. The individual or the group decides the word they want to use as their intention for the day. At the conclusion of the day's Experiential Therapy activity in nature, that word is revisited and discussed in terms of how it influenced their thinking, process, awareness in nature, and emotions during the activity.

One Experiential Therapist, Susan Foster, has created a photo album of pictures of the particular trail that clients will be on with her. The clients can peruse the photo album prior to beginning the hike so that they are familiar with what they may expect to see on the trail (personal communication, June 3, 2023). Foster has found that this allays the fears and anxiety of clients who have very limited or no experience being in nature. It is a preview of what to expect.

Metaphors in Nature

The natural environment also gives us some great metaphors that we can use to help reinforce the conversations we are having. For instance, when looking at a tree we can discuss: *roots* (where they came from, who were the important people in their lives when they were growing up, what nourishes them, what and who helps them grow), *trunks* (what makes them strong, what and who holds them up, how they can be flexible to bend with the wind but not break), *branches* (what are the many paths they have taken in life, when have they broken off branches that no longer served them or were no longer stable for them, when have they needed to return to a more solid part of the tree again), and *leaves* (the seasons of leaves: the leaves growing from tendrils—what are the early memories of their lives; the changing colors of leaves—the discussion of their development; leaves falling—releasing what they no longer need or what is no longer helpful to them; and cycling through another season to increased growth, development, awareness, and resilience). Additionally, trees in winter, though perceived as not living, are just waiting for the spring to revive themselves and start anew, which is great for folks who are at a crossroads and need time to consider which way to proceed.

Other metaphors can come from the weather or the time of the day. For instance, *sunshine* (what warms them, gives them joy, makes them happy, helps them see more clearly), *wind* (what cools them when they feel overheated, what causes destruction for them if the wind is strong; but also a strong wind can be used to ask what they need to do to clean out the old and make space for the new), *rain* (what dashes hopes and dreams for the moment for them, but conversely can be used to ask what nurtures them and gives them sustenance, and how can they comfortably pause and change direction if rain changes their plans), and *darkness* (what keeps them from being able to fully see or be aware of what is actually helping in their lives, what scares them or makes them wary of change or growth).

Additionally, particular natural phenomena that you come across in nature are also great metaphors and teachable moments. For instance, when you look at a body of water, a creek, a river, a lake, or an ocean, is it clear and calm where you can see your own reflection and deep into the depths, or is it churned up and you cannot see your reflection or what lies beneath? The calm versus turbulent waters is a great metaphor for couples and families of when to discuss important issues so that people can be heard, listened to, understood, and comprehended, and solutions can be found. It also gives insight into when a situation is escalating, it is not the right time to enter water that has been churned up and the bottom cannot be seen. There are times for discussion and times to separate until the water can be restored to its calm state.

Rocks can also create great metaphors. The persistence, immovability, and continuity of large rocks and boulders can be used to discuss barriers in their lives that, even though they would like them to go away, are long-standing and need to be circumvented or climbed over. Either going around or going over will take time, energy, persistence, and determination, but can be overcome. Conversely, rocks in water can be discussed as the wearing down of rocks, making them less rough, less pointed, and smaller in size and more easily traversable. This can be a helpful metaphor in the process of trauma therapy in that through therapy the roughness, pointedness, and inability to pass by the rock has changed; it is no longer such an impediment for forward movement. The striations of rocks can also be discussed as relating to each individual's unique qualities and beauty, especially when they are more closely examined—just as people, when you take the time to know them, are uniquely beautiful and interesting. Additionally, one can often find rocks that have plants growing through them, which are great symbols of resilience and persistence.

Depending on the ecosystem where you live, there are literally thousands of metaphors that can be used, such as *acorns* (how can such a tiny seed turn into a magnificent oak tree?), or *prickly pear cactus* (how can a barbed plant have such a sweet fruit?). Why do *lichen* grow around the entire tree, while *moss* only grows on the north side of a tree? These are opportunities to discuss, ponder, and see how they relate to clients in particular bioregions.

Knowledge of Your Bioregion

A noted clinician and founder of the Colorado Ecotherapy Institute (http://www.coloradoecotherapyinstitute.com), Kimberly Rose (personal communication, May 31, 2023) suggests that to do therapy in nature, the clinician needs to have some basic competency in nature knowledge and awareness, that the love of nature is not enough. The clinician should know the bioregion where they will be doing therapy. Rose suggests that the clinician learn to recognize the significant trees, poisonous plants, medicinal plants, birds, insects, invasive plants, and animal tracks found in the area. By studying these dwellers of the natural world, the client can better understand the protective strategies of plants (hairs, thorns, prickles, and volatile oils) to help similarly understand one's own protective strategies, defensive strategies, and methods of increasing one's own survival, well-being, and resilience.

Rose sees bringing clients outdoors as an opportunity for clients to build or rebuild a relationship with the natural environment, which is a relationship that many have neglected. Rose believes that all therapy at its root is helping the client connect to and better understand all their relationships. Thus, therapy in nature is helping the client pay attention to their nourishing relationship with nature and simultaneously how to better establish the important relationships in their lives.

Creating Awe

A new science is emerging, the science of "awe" (Keltner, 2024). It has been described as "being amazed at the things outside of ourselves" and is being scientifically studied (Keltner, 2024, p. xxvi). It has been evaluated that by creating awe in our own lives, we can greatly improve the quality of our lives, our health, and well-being (Keltner, 2024). One of the greatest places for creating awe is nature: looking at stars in the night sky, mountains, canyons, large trees, sand dunes, oceans, new plants breaking through the soil, insects moving objects twice their size, the poise of a wild animal, and so on. It gives us a sense of wonder that what we are experiencing is larger than ourselves (Keltner, 2024). Thus, bringing clients into nature helps them connect and feel awe at the enormity of the mountain or the complexity of a spider web. Awe helps individuals realize that we are part of the natural world and interdependent upon each other for survival (Keltner, 2024). By doing so, awe helps support and protect the natural environment and simultaneously helps support our best growth and development. When we bring clients into the natural environment, we can often create experiences of awe for them, which they can later reflect upon, and this gives us many clinical segues.

Soloing

Another activity you may want to have your clients try is soloing. Soloing is the opportunity for the client to sit quietly in nature and reflect for a little while on their own. This is not an activity to do in their first visits in nature, but once they feel more comfortable in nature.

First, you need to explain that sitting quietly in nature may help them collect their thoughts and help them gain new insight into old issues. It is an opportunity to be still, to be aware of their surroundings, to listen to the sounds of the wind, birds, insects, grass, trees, and themselves. It is an opportunity be an observer. The first time they try this, you should set an alarm for 10 minutes and they should stay in close enough proximity to you that they can see you. Over time, if they enjoy the activity, they can extend their time soloing up to an hour. As they venture farther afield, you may want to carry a boat foghorn with you since your voice may not be heard at a greater distance to call them back.

While they are soloing, they may want to bring with them a camera, binoculars, a cushion to sit on, a journal and writing utensils, or art supplies. Some clients will find soloing to be an opportunity for meditation. You can promote this meditation by using a word such as "roots, clear, open, shine, grateful, flow, connect, spirit, still" (Grasse, 2023, pp. 5–6) to begin their meditative process.

Some will find that this time in nature increases their connection to their creative selves and may want to do artwork in nature. Others may find that this time of quiet reflection is an opportunity to put their thoughts on paper and journal about their thoughts or their experience in nature. Others will simply enjoy relaxing in nature.

Some will want to better view what is happening around them and use binoculars to better see the plants and animals in their midst. Kimberly Rose has clients listen to and view the birds around them alerting others when people enter an area, and then listen for the birds to go silent and after a bit begin to chirp to each other again. She calls this a "bird break"—a pause to assess the new intruders in their midst, before returning to communicating again. The metaphor of the bird break can be used in many ways of taking a pause, and waiting to see what happens before proceeding again.

Once clients return from soloing, they often have a lot to say about what they thought about, what they observed, and the connections they made in nature. Often you can visibly see a new calmness on their face and in their bodies. It affords the ability to create clinical segues of what they gained through soloing and how to connect that to other spheres of their lives.

Progression of Experiential in Nature Activities

It is important to slowly offer new outdoor activities over time if clients would like to try new things, being mindful that before leveling up to a more "off the grid" or more rugged activity, it is necessary to ensure that they are ready (both physically and mentally) to do so. Remember that it is always challenge by choice. The client may prefer to sit with you on a bench in a city park for several weeks, or even the duration of the therapy. Movement from a bench sit, to a park walk, to sitting at trailhead, to hiking on the trail, to increasing the duration of the hike, or snowshoeing, or using a new hiking venue or snowshoeing destination are all a slow and deliberate process to keep the client in the learning zone and not the panic zone.

Experiential Therapy in Nature Protocols by Season

We are sharing with you a variety of nature-based Experiential Therapy protocols. We hand these protocols out for the specific outdoor activity and discuss them with clients prior to their being involved in the outdoor activity. We have found that by having these protocols, it increases their knowledge of the outdoor activity, their responsibilities in the natural environment, and reduces risks for clients as well as ourselves. We have organized them by season and by low to higher risk.

Throughout the Year

Walk Protocol

Expected Time: 1+ hours

Purpose/Objective: To use a walk as a tool for doing Experiential Therapy. We will be walking at [NAME OF PARK]. We will meet at the [EXACT LOCATION] at the Park.

Age, Gender, Physical Ability, and Cultural Considerations:

- Need parental consent if under 18.

- Need to be healthy to be involved in this cardio activity; get medical approval prior to being involved.

Equipment/Materials Needed:

- Clothing: shorts/pants (depending on time of year and weather)
- T-shirt
- Insulated jacket (if cooler) and rain jacket
- Socks
- Hiking boots or athletic shoes
- Sunglasses
- Water bottle
- Snacks as needed
- Suntan lotion
- Backpack if desired but not necessary.
- MUST HAVE APPROPRIATE CLOSED-TOE FOOTWEAR
- MUST HAVE WATER BOTTLE

Disclaimer: If the client does NOT wear appropriate attire and have good working equipment per the therapist's estimation, she/he/they will not be able to participate in the activity.

Risk Assessment: Need to be healthy to participate in this activity; get doctor's approval

Risks You May Be Exposed to:

- Allergies/asthma (bring meds or inhaler if necessary)
- Injury (therapist will have first aid kit; however, if there is a fall, medical care may be needed)
- Unpredictability of nature—weather, wildlife, terrain, sunburn

How to Best Prepare Yourself for This Activity

What Not to Bring:

- No animals
- No drugs/alcohol
- No weapons
- No tobacco (no nicotine products, including vaping)

Check the weather before the session.
If you have any questions, feel free to contact the therapist before the activity.
Be aware of road conditions on your way to the activity, as well.

Hiking Protocol

Expected Time: 1+ hours

Purpose/Objective: To use hiking as a tool for doing Experiential Therapy. We will be hiking at [NAME OF TRAILHEAD or PARK]. We will meet at the [EXACT LOCATION] at the Trailhead/Park.

Age, Gender, Physical Ability, and Cultural Considerations:

- Need parental consent if under 18.
- Need to be healthy to be involved in this cardio activity; get medical approval prior to being involved.

Equipment/Materials Needed:

- Clothing: shorts/pants (Depending on time of year and weather)
- T-shirt
- Insulated jacket (if cooler) and rain jacket
- Socks
- Hiking boots or athletic shoes
- Sunglasses
- Water bottle
- Snacks as needed
- Sunscreen lotion
- Backpack if desired but not necessary
- MUST HAVE APPROPRIATE CLOSED-TOE FOOTWEAR
- MUST HAVE WATER BOTTLE

Disclaimer: If the client does NOT wear appropriate attire and have good working equipment per therapist's estimation, she/he/they will not be able to participate in the activity.

Risk Assessment: Need to be healthy to participate in this activity; get doctor's approval.

Risks You May Be Exposed to:

- Allergies/asthma (bring meds or inhaler if necessary)
- Injury (therapist will have first aid kit; however, if there is a fall, medical care may be needed)
- Unpredictability of nature—weather, wildlife, terrain, sunburn

How to Best Prepare Yourself for This Activity

What Not to Bring:

- No animals

- No drugs/alcohol
- No weapons
- No tobacco (no nicotine products, including vaping)

Check the weather before the session.

If you have any questions, feel free to contact the therapist before the activity.

Be aware of road conditions on your way to the activity, as well.

Spring, Summer, and Fall

Challenge Course Protocol

Expected Time: 4–8 hours

Purpose/Objective: To use the challenge course as a tool for doing Experiential Therapy. Ground, Low, and High Elements are offered in a challenge by choice philosophy with family/partner/group and clinician. The "hard skills" will be provided by the Licensed Challenge Course Organization. We will be going to the Challenge Course at [NAME OF CHALLENGE COURSE]. We will meet at the [EXACT LOCATION] at the Challenge Course.

Age, Gender, Physical Ability, and Cultural Considerations:

- Need parental consent if under 18.
- Need to be healthy to be involved in this activity; get medical approval prior to being involved.

Equipment/Materials Needed:

- Clothing: shorts/pants, T-shirt, jacket, rain jacket
- Socks (2 pair)
- Medications (if needed)
- Shoes (athletic shoes or hiking boots; NO SANDALS OR OPEN-TOE SHOES)
- Sunglasses
- Gloves/hat/visor
- Water in water bottle
- Snacks as needed
- Lunch (there is no refrigeration)
- Sunscreen

What Will Be Provided for You:

- Water

Disclaimer: If the client does NOT wear appropriate attire and have good working equipment per therapist's estimation, she/he/they will not be able to participate in the activity.

Risk Assessment: Need to be healthy to participate in this activity; get doctor's approval.

Risks You May Be Exposed to:

- Allergies/asthma (bring meds or inhaler if necessary)
- Injury (therapist will have first aid kit; however, if there is a fall, medical care may be needed)
- Unpredictability of nature—weather, wildlife, terrain, sunburn

How to Best Prepare Yourself for This Activity:

What Not to Bring:

- No animals
- No drugs/alcohol
- No weapons
- No tobacco (no nicotine products, including vaping)

Check the weather before the session.
If you have any questions, feel free to contact the therapist before the activity.
Be aware of road conditions on your way to the activity, as well.

Road Biking Protocol

Expected Time: 1+ hours

Purpose/Objective: To use biking as a tool for doing Experiential Therapy. This is not a training ride but a leisure ride where we can talk throughout. We will be biking at [NAME OF PARK]. We will meet at the [EXACT LOCATION] at the Park.

Age, Gender, Physical Ability, and Cultural Considerations:

- Need parental consent if under 18.
- Need to be healthy to be involved in this cardio activity; get medical approval prior to being involved.

Equipment/Materials Needed for Biking:

- Clothing: bike shorts, T-shirt, jacket (if cooler)
- Socks

- Shoes (athletic shoes or bike shoes)
- Sunglasses
- Gloves (if desired)
- MUST HAVE HELMET
- MUST HAVE BIKE
- Water in water bottle that fits on your bike OR water in backpack
- Snacks as needed
- Sunscreen lotion

What Will Be Provided for You:

- You will need to bring your own bike and helmet, we will NOT be providing any equipment.

Disclaimer: If the client does NOT wear appropriate attire and have good working equipment per therapist's estimation, she/he/they will not be able to participate in the activity.

Risk Assessment:

- Need to be able to ride a bike.
- Need to be healthy to participate in this cardio activity; get medical approval.

Risks You May Be Exposed to:

- Allergies/asthma (bring meds or inhaler if necessary)
- Injury (therapist will have first aid kit; however, if there is a fall, medical care may be needed)
- Unpredictability of nature—weather, wildlife, terrain, sunburn

How to Best Prepare Yourself for This Activity:

What Not to Bring:

- No animals
- No drugs/alcohol
- No weapons
- No tobacco (no nicotine products, including vaping)

Check the weather before the session.
If you have any questions, feel free to contact the therapist before the activity.
Be aware of road conditions on your way to the activity, as well.

Summer Only

Camping Protocol

Expected Time: 24 hours

Purpose/Objective: To use camping as a tool for doing Experiential Therapy. This is not a survival activity, but an opportunity to spend time in nature with family/partner/group and clinician. We will be camping at the [NAME OF PARK]. We will meet at the [EXACT LOCATION] of the Park.

Age, Gender, Physical Ability, and Cultural Considerations:

- Need parental consent if under 18.
- Need to be healthy to be involved in this overnight activity, get medical approval prior to being involved.

Equipment/Materials Needed:

- Clothing: shorts/pants, T-shirts, jacket, rain jacket, sleeping attire
- Socks (2 pair)
- Shoes (athletic shoes or hiking boots)
- Sunglasses
- Gloves/hat
- Headlamp
- Sleeping bag and pillow
- Water in water bottle
- Snacks as needed
- Sunscreen
- Camping chair
- Plate, cup, and utensils
- Any medications you take
- Electric lantern (if desired)
- Food: (1) discuss dietary restrictions; (2) create menus prior to camping; (3) decide who will be bringing what food.

What Will Be Provided for You:

- Tent and camping equipment from a reputable rental company.
- Cooking stove, cooking utensils, and fire starter from a reputable rental company.
- Garbage bags

Disclaimer: If the client does NOT wear appropriate attire and have good working equipment per therapist's estimation, she/he/they will not be able to participate in the activity.

Risk Assessment:

- Need to be able to spend night outdoors.
- Need to be healthy to participate in this activity; get medical approval.

Risks You May Be Exposed to:

- Allergies/asthma (bring meds or inhaler if necessary)
- Injury (therapist will have first aid kit; however, if there is a fall, medical care may be needed)
- Unpredictability of nature—weather, wildlife, terrain, sunburn

How to Best Prepare Yourself for This Activity:

What Not to Bring:

- No animals
- No drugs/alcohol
- No weapons
- No tobacco (no nicotine products, including vaping)

Check the weather before the session.
If you have any questions, feel free to contact the therapist before the activity.
Be aware of road conditions on your way to the activity, as well.

Paddleboarding Protocol

Expected Time: 1+hours

Purpose/Objective: To use paddleboarding as a tool for doing Experiential Therapy. We will be paddleboarding at [NAME OF PARK]. We will meet at the [EXACT LOCATION] in the Park.

Age, Gender, Physical Ability, and Cultural Considerations:

- Need parental consent if under 18; must be 10 years old or older.
- Need to be healthy to be involved in this cardio activity; get medical approval prior to being involved.

- Need to know how to swim.
- You will need to wear the provided life preserver for the entire activity.

Equipment/Materials Needed:

- Swimsuit
- Sunglasses (if desired); make sure they have a strap, so you don't lose them
- Sunscreen

What Will Be Provided for You:

- Paddleboard, paddle, and life preserver from licensed paddle rental at park.

Disclaimer: If the client does NOT wear appropriate attire and have good working equipment per therapist's estimation, she/he/they will not be able to participate in the activity.

Risk Assessment: Need to be healthy to participate in this activity; get medical approval.

Risks You May Be Exposed to:

- Allergies/asthma (bring meds or inhaler if necessary)
- Injury (therapist will have first aid kit; however, if there is a fall, medical care may be needed)
- Unpredictability of nature—weather, wildlife, terrain, sunburn

How to Best Prepare Yourself for This Activity:

What Not to Bring:

- No animals
- No drugs/alcohol
- No weapons
- No tobacco (no nicotine products, including vaping)

Check the weather before the session.
If you have any questions, feel free to contact the therapist before the activity.
Be aware of road conditions on your way to the activity, as well.

Winter Only

Snowshoeing Protocol

Expected Time: 1+ hour

Purpose/Objective: To use snowshoeing as a tool for doing Experiential Therapy. We will be snowshoeing at [NAME OF PARK]. We will meet at the [EXACT LOCATION] in the Park. *Age, Gender, Physical Ability, and Cultural Considerations*:

- Need parental consent if under 18 and must be 10 years old or older.
- Need to be healthy to be involved in this cardio activity; get medical approval prior to being involved.

Equipment/Materials Needed:

- Clothing: winter jacket, snow pants, hat, and gloves/mittens
- Base layer
- Long johns
- Waterproof and insulated boots
- Warm socks
- Extra pair of warm socks
- Sunglasses (if desired)
- Face mask or scarf (if desired)
- Backpack (if desired)
- MUST HAVE PROPER COLD WEATHER GEAR AND FOOTWEAR
- Water in water bottle OR water in backpack
- Snacks as needed
- Sunscreen

What Will Be Provided for You:

- Snowshoes rented from a reputable vendor.

Disclaimer: If the client does NOT wear appropriate attire and have good working equipment per therapist's estimation, she/he/they will not be able to participate in the activity.

Risk Assessment: Need to be healthy to participate in this activity; get medical approval.

Risks you may be exposed to:

- Allergies/asthma (bring meds or inhaler if necessary)
- Injury (therapist will have first aid kit; however, if there is a fall, medical care may be needed)
- Unpredictability of nature—weather, wildlife, terrain, sunburn

How to Best Prepare Yourself for This Activity:

What Not to Bring:

- No animals
- No drugs/alcohol
- No weapons
- No tobacco (no nicotine products, including vaping)

Check the weather before the session.

If you have any questions, feel free to contact the therapist before the activity.

Be aware of road conditions on your way to the activity, as well.

These are protocols we regularly use in Colorado. You will need to modify them for your own bioregion. However, it gives you the important elements that you need to share with your clients. Happy trails to you!

Next Chapter

In Chapter 9, we will discuss Experiential Therapy in the virtual realm.

Chapter 9
Experiential Therapy in the Virtual Realm

When the world closed down completely due to COVID-19, we had to rework how we were delivering Experiential Therapy. It took some time to understand how to convert and maintain clinical relationships in an online platform. Some activities were impossible to do online, but many, with a little creativity, would have a very similar effect. One benefit we found was that it also gave us opportunities to work with clients who did not live in our community. We also learned how to effectively move our business to an online platform, which also took time and understanding the rules of the virtual world. We would like to share with you this information. At the end of the chapter, we will share three virtual Experiential Therapy activities and a virtual walk.

Lessons Learned for Best Practice in a Virtual World

HIPAA Compliant Platform

First of all, not all online platforms are HIPAA (the Health Insurance Portability and Accountability Act, ensuring that individuals' health information is properly protected) compliant platforms. This means that some online platforms we use regularly do not meet the stringent standards of protecting clients' information. Make sure the online platform you are planning to use is HIPAA compliant. If you are unsure, send them an email to verify.

Confidentiality

Confidentiality becomes much more of an issue when you are seeing clients online. Since clients aren't seeing you in your office or outside together where

Understanding and Effectively Utilizing Experiential Therapy. Julie Anne Laser and Nicole Nicotera,
Oxford University Press. © Oxford University Press (2025). DOI: 10.1093/9780197757581.003.0009

you can monitor who is in the area, you cannot completely protect their confidentiality on their end. For instance, there may be someone listening in to the conversation who is off screen or in an adjacent room. Thus, this may create a scenario in which the client may not feel comfortable speaking about issues that involve the other people who may be listening, or the client may feel they need to avoid certain topics or put topics in a different light because other people may be listening in.

You will need to assist them to find ways they can increase their own confidentiality. It is recommended that the client be in a quiet place, preferably wearing headphones so that they can hear us clearly and others cannot, with a closed and preferably locked door so others do not inadvertently wander into the room.

Some clients may prefer to hold the appointment outside. Some clients sat in their garden or in their backyard for therapy. Some clients felt most at ease to take their appointment in the car; some would just sit in their car in their garage or driveway and others would drive to a pretty place to park and look out while online. The point is that there are always workarounds that give the clients the flexibility they need, so that they feel that it is always challenge by choice and they can still maintain confidentiality.

Practicing

When COVID-19 closed everything down, there were many clinicians who began seeing clients throughout the country, not just in their community. However, to do this legally, the therapist needs to hold a license in every state where a client resides. Thus, we have one colleague who holds licenses in 27 states. This is both a major endeavor and a major expenditure. However, some clinicians have enjoyed connecting with a much broader community. There is also legislation pending that some states will offer interstate compacts in the future.

Connectivity

You should create a protocol for your practice and share that information with your clients, including what the procedure is if internet connectivity is lost during a session. For instance, living in the Colorado foothills, it is not uncommon for us that internet becomes unstable, or we lose connectivity when we have big snowstorms. We needed to make a plan of what we would do when the internet drops when we are with a client and also what we would do if the internet was down for a longer period of time and our next clients would also be offline. We found that we should always have an alternate way to complete the session and share that information with our clients prior to issues developing. For us, we needed to make sure we had our clients' cell phone numbers, and that they were available and willing, if needed, to finish a session by cell phone or text or to have a session by cell phone or text if necessary due to the internet instability. Additionally, on days when we are supposed to get a lot of snow, we need to remind the client at the beginning of the session of the alternative plan if we lose internet connectivity.

Payment

Payment online is much easier than it has been before and there are a variety of sites that accept credit card payments that put the funds into your account, or direct deposits are possible from many clients' banks to your bank now. However, you need to discuss payment for sessions and how payment will be made when they first sign up for counseling. We have found that it is much easier to set the ground rules and the expectations for payment prior to their beginning therapy.

Cancellation Policy

One of the issues that can be frustrating and sometimes even financially deleterious are clients canceling or not showing up for appointments. We have a 24-hour cancellation policy which spells out that if they do not contact us 24 hours prior to their appointment we will charge them whether or not they attend the appointment. Make sure your cancellation policy is written out in your initial materials you send to the client and on your website, and also is verbally stated to the client. This is a proactive measure that can avoid a lot of headaches when a cancellation or a no-show does occur. Obviously, if they are having an emergency, then allowances can be made. But having a stated cancellation policy means that you can count on having clients present at agreed-upon times. Additionally, it can help move wait-listed clients into appointments sooner if you know in advance a client will not be attending a session. It also supports your own financial viability by knowing that the hours you plan to work will be paid hours.

Emergencies

It is important to consider what your policy is in case of client emergencies. Remember, if you are doing virtual Experiential Therapy with a client out of your area code and you call 911, the emergency operator will not be able to help your client. It is important to get the telephone number of the local Psychiatric Emergency Room, Emergency Room, and Police Department where your client is situated for EVERY virtual client and to know the address where they plan to be physically located during sessions, so that when you speak to emergency personnel you know where to send them. It is also highly recommended to have an emergency contact telephone number and person for EACH client. You should discuss with your client that the emergency contact person should be someone with whom they would be comfortable for you breaking confidentiality. The client should understand that this would only be done in an emergency, but that having someone near their actual location could be extremely beneficial.

Consent to Treat

Review the consent form with the client and have them sign it electronically (docu-sign or similar online signature) and send it back electronically to have a copy in their file. If they are uncomfortable or unwilling to use an online signature, you will need to send them the documents through the mail and not begin sessions until you receive the returned signed copy. Never begin therapy until you have the necessary forms in place.

Virtual Experiential Therapy Activities

We have included a few Experiential Therapy activities that work particularly well online. We are continually creating new virtual activities and trying to reinvent our face-to-face activities for the virtual realm.

Virtual Scavenger Hunt

Time Duration: 15 minutes to 1 hour, depending on number of clients and the stories elicited from the objects

Purpose/Objective: To create symbols of yourself and your journey through life

Age/Gender/Cultural Considerations: As long as they can gather items on their own, they can do this activity. Appropriate for any gender.

Equipment/Materials Needed: Items that have a symbolic value. If they do not have the item in their possession, a picture of that item would work, or they could draw a picture of it.

Risk Assessment: The biggest issue is to make sure they are comfortable sharing that item with you or the group. Remind them that drug paraphernalia and weapons are not appropriate.

Framing Question: What symbols do you hold on to that represent your past, present, and future?

Directions for Activity:

1. Explain that you are giving each of them X minutes of time.
2. Tell them that this is a silent activity until they come back to the group and are asked to share.
3. Tell them they will need to find three things.
4. First, ask them to find an object that reminds them of their past selves. If they don't have the object, they can use their cell phone or computer to find a picture of the item or show a past picture. If they don't have a cell phone, they could draw a picture of it.
5. Then they need to sit and look at it for a bit and consider what reminds them of their past selves. What are the characteristics of the object? Why is it important for them? Why do they see themselves that way?
6. Second, ask them to find another object that represents their current selves and go through the same process of gathering it, or finding a picture of it or drawing it, and then contemplating: What are the characteristics of the object? Why is it important for them? Why do they see their current self that way?
7. Then third, they need to find an object that is how they want to see themselves in the future and go through the same process of gathering it, or finding a picture of it or drawing it, and then considering: What are the characteristics of the object? Why is it important for them? Why do they see their future selves that way?

8. Tell them that when the time is up, they will come back together and share (if they want to share, as it is challenge by choice) their objects or pictures/artwork with the group.

9. Have the group all share their past item first, explaining what it is and why it is important to them.

10. Then, when all who have wanted to share their past item have done so, ask all who want to share their present item with the group, explaining what it is and why it is important to them.

11. Finally, when all who have wanted to share their present item have done so, ask them to share their future item with the group, explaining what it is and why it is important to them.

Clinical Segues and Questions:

- How was it to find objects that represented themselves?
- Was this easy or difficult?
- What did you learn about yourself doing the activity?
- What did you learn about your journey through life?
- How do you envision your future?
- How did hearing and seeing other people's objects affect you?
- Did you learn more about your group members?
- In the future, when you are feeling activated or having a tough day, can you use these objects or pictures of these objects to support to you?

For Whom Would This Activity Be Appropriate, and for Whom Would It Not Be Appropriate?

As long as the group members have mobility to gather the objects or draw, this will work well.

Who Is It? (Virtual)

Time Duration: 20–40 minutes, depending on size of group

Purpose/Objective: Remembering and learning new things about each other

Age/Gender/Cultural Considerations: Appropriate for children about 8 years old and up; appropriate for any gender.

Equipment/Materials Needed: none

Risk Assessment: Low to medium, challenge by choice: participants can choose how much or how little personal information they share; remind them that substance use, sexual escapades, and illegal behavior are not discussed.

Framing Questions: Let's see what we can remember about those in our group and how much we take in. We have spent time with this group for X sessions. What have we learned about each other?

Directions for Activity:

1. Each group member privately messages the facilitator three facts about themselves. This can include favorites, such as food, color, or movie; places they have visited or lived; things they have done; or any other interesting facts.
2. Share examples about different facts that can be used, such as: I like to go skiing; my favorite food is pizza; I was born in Wisconsin. This can be helpful for younger participants.
3. The clinician will let the group know when they have received a private message from each participant.
4. The clinician will read out one fact at a time, pausing between facts to give group members time to guess who the person is.
5. Each group member gets one guess.
6. If the group member is not guessed by the time everyone's guess is used, the clinician tells the group who it is.
7. Once the person is guessed successfully or the clinician tells who it was to the group, the information about the next person is read by the clinician until everyone's information has been shared.

Clinical Segues and Questions:

- How did it feel to have your information read out loud?
- How did it feel for people to guess it was you right away?
- Or did they think it was someone else first? How did that feel?
- Did you know the identity of the person the information was describing right away?
- Or did it take you a long time to figure out who was being described?
- How observant are we?
- How good are we at listening?
- How can we become more observant?
- How can we be better listeners?
- Are we ever upset with people who do not pay attention to us? Or listen to us? Or do not really see us?

For Whom Would This Activity Be Appropriate, and for Whom Would It Not Be Appropriate?
   If group members have lots of anxiety, this may be stressful, even though they may be very good observers and guessers as to who it is. The group must have had several sessions together so that they know something about each other.

Xerox or Partner Draw (Virtual)

Time duration: 15 minutes

Purpose/Objective: To discover the complexity of precise communication

Age/Gender/Cultural Considerations: Participants need to be able to use a writing utensil and know shapes.

Equipment/Materials Needed: One piece of paper and a writing utensil for each partner

Risk Assessment: Minimal risk

Framing Question: How do we effectively communicate with each other so that the other person understands what we are saying?

Directions for Activity:

1. Each partner gets a piece of paper, a writing utensil, and a surface to write on (e.g., a clipboard, a book).
2. Sit so that you cannot see the other person's paper on the screen. If there are many pairs, then they need to be sent to breakout rooms.
3. Decide who will draw the original first.
4. Then one partner, the original drawer, draws five shapes on the paper.
5. The original drawer describes to the Xerox drawer what is on the paper: location, shape, and size. (For more challenge, the Xerox drawer can only ask yes or no questions of the original drawer. The original drawer can only answer yes or no.)
6. Share the results. Repeat with changing roles of original drawer and Xerox drawer.

Clinical Segues and Questions:

- How closely do the two pictures resemble one another?
- How important was it for you to be precise about your language?
- What feelings did this bring up for you?
- How do you communicate normally? Is it effective communication?
- Can this help you to be a better communicator in the future?

- How could you have understood better what your partner was saying?
- Do you have trouble understanding what each other is saying in other venues in your life?
- How can you better communicate with each other?

For Whom Would This Activity Be Appropriate, and for Whom Would It Not Be Appropriate?
This works well with most couples. It can also be a great assessment tool to better understand how they communicate with each other. If the couple is very argumentative, you may want them only to be able to use yes/no questions at first. This also works well with families, children over about age 8, and youth. This activity would need to be modified for people who are hearing impaired. It may not work for people who are vison impaired.

Virtual Walks

We continued during COVID-19 lockdown to walk with some of our clients, via online platforms. We would start from our house and walk in our neighborhood, and they would start from their home and walk in their own neighborhood. We had to be especially careful about "dead zone" internet areas on walks. It was not the same, but it was close, and it got people out of the house and into the fresh air.

Next Chapter

In Chapter 10, we discuss Experiential Therapy activities with specific populations: children, youth, couples, and families.

Chapter 10
Experiential Therapy Activities With Specific Populations

In this chapter, we are sharing with you a lot of Experiential Therapy activities that have been used successfully with many populations, but we have categorized them under specific populations to give you transferable skills right away for whatever population you are working with. We have separated them by age, giving you interventions for both children and youth, and by family organization by couples and families. With most of these interventions, they can be easily transferred to a different population with minimal or no modifications. We felt this gives you a wide repertoire of Experiential Therapy activities to use right away in your practice.

Children

Doing Experiential therapy with children is a fun, active way of doing clinical work. Children usually join in almost immediately since for them they see it as play and not an intense clinical experience. Children can be great sources of support for each other, if they are encouraged to show their best selves. Experiential Therapy provides an opportunity for group members to let their guard down, play, communicate, and grow. By engaging children in Experiential Therapy activities, they gain both a greater sense of self and knowledge of others.

For children, Experiential Therapy is also a great assessment tool because almost from the start, they show up as themselves and are not trying to present as a version of themselves. Thus, we can see how they interact with each other, how they listen, how they express themselves, how they deal with frustration, their level of curiosity, their level of willingness to try new things, their level of social anxiety, and their stick-to-it-ness. With older elementary school–aged children, they can often make the clinical segues themselves. For younger children, we like to call it a "teachable moment" where we as the Experiential Therapists can help them bridge the Experiential Therapy activity to their "real" life.

Understanding and Effectively Utilizing Experiential Therapy. Julie Anne Laser and Nicole Nicotera,
Oxford University Press. © Oxford University Press (2025). DOI: 10.1093/9780197757581.003.0010

Blind Polygon

Time Duration: 10–30 minutes

Purpose/Objective: This activity encourages groups to work on effective communication, collaboration, team strategy, and problem-solving.

Age/Gender/Cultural Considerations: It can be used with nearly any group. Adaptations may be needed for younger children or individuals with disabilities. This can be a very frustrating activity, so adjust the level of difficulty based on the needs of the group. It is appropriate for any gender.

Equipment/Materials Needed: One blindfold/bandana for every participant, 20–40 feet of rope or string, depending on group size.

Risk Assessment: Low risk. However, the activity does call for individuals to be blind-folded, so address this aspect in the framing and allow participants through challenge by choice to use a blindfold or not. Due to the fact that they're blindfolded, ensure that the group performs the activity in a flat, obstacle-free space so as to prevent injury from falls.

Framing Question: You will be asked to work as a group to create a certain shape using the rope/string provided. Both your hands must remain on the rope/string at all times once the activity begins. Please keep your blindfolds on until the group agrees the task is complete.

Directions for Activity:

1. Ask the group to form a circle.
2. Once in place, ask the group to put their blindfolds on; those who do not want to wear a blindfold must agree to keep their eyes closed.
3. Ask the group members to have their hands outstretched.
4. Carefully place the rope in each member's hands.
5. Ask the group to form a triangle.
6. Once they collectively agree that they've completed their task, they may take their blindfolds off, or open their eyes, to see how close they were at creating a triangle.
7. You can do the activity as many times as the group desires, using different shapes such as square, rectangle, circle, diamond, or oval. If they would like and you have a large enough group, they can make shapes like pentagon, octagon, heart, or star.

Clinical Segues and Questions:
   How did you most effectively work together?

Did a leader or leaders emerge?

What was the most challenging aspect of this activity?

How did the group deal with frustration?

How did you deal with frustration?

How did it feel to see the shape you created?

Were you proud of what you created?

For Whom Would This Activity Be Appropriate, and for Whom Would It Not Be Appropriate?

This activity works with most people. Some individuals really do not like wearing a blindfold, so make sure that they do not feel they need to wear one if it is activating for them.

A Tangled Web

Time Duration:10–30 minutes

Purpose/Objective: This is an activity that helps us to further learn about each other.

Age/Gender/Cultural Considerations: Appropriate for children and up; appropriate for any gender.

Equipment/Materials Needed: Large ball of yarn or thin rope

Risk Assessment: Low to medium risk. Remind group members about challenge by choice; participants can choose how much or how little personal information they share. Once again, remind them that substance use, sexual escapades, and illegal behavior are not discussed.

Framing Question: What do we share in common and what sets us apart?

Directions for Activity:

1. Ask the group to sit/stand in a circle.
2. Inform group members that if they are uncomfortable answering a question, they can "pass" and throw the ball of yarn back to the group member who asked the question and was previously holding it to ask them a new question.
3. The first person with the ball of yarn throws the ball to another group member.
4. The thrower of the yarn asks the catcher of the yarn a question, such as: Where were you born? What's your favorite food? What's the last book/movie you

read/saw? How long have you lived here? What's the hardest thing you've ever done? What's one thing you really like about yourself? If you could go anywhere in the world, where would you go? If you could be any kind of animal, what would it be and why? If you could be anything when you grow up, what would you be? What is your best quality? What has been your happiest day? What has been your saddest day? When were you most proud of yourself? Who do you look up to?

5. The receiver of the ball of yarn then shares their response, remembering that if they do not want to answer they can throw the ball back and ask for a new question.
6. While holding on to the yarn, the responder then rolls or throws the ball to a different group member, and the process is repeated until everyone has had a chance to answer a question.
7. This can continue as many times as time allows.
8. The web will get thicker and more complex the more times the ball travels around the circle.
9. With everyone holding on to the yarn/string, have them hold the web up overhead. The web should still be strong and complex.
10. Have one person drop their yarn. What happened to the web?
11. Then have another, and another, until the yarn is on the ground.

Clinical Segues and Questions:
    What did you learn about each other?
    What were some surprises you found out about others?
    What's it like to be part of a group where not everyone is the same?
    Did you feel sympathy/empathy (explain these terms) for other group members?
    Can you relate to other group members because of the activity?
    We are all similar and we are all unique, aren't we?
    What happens when one group member dropped their strand? How does this relate to teamwork?
    We are all needed in this group to make it a success, aren't we?
    For Whom Would This Activity Be Appropriate, and for Whom Would It Not Be Appropriate?

This is a good activity once the group has met a few times. They need to be far enough along in group development that they feel they can be vulnerable enough to answer the questions from each other.

Passing the Paper

Time Duration: 20–30 minutes

Purpose/Objective: To help encourage and bring positive energy into each group member's life. This is often used as a closing activity for the group. It also creates something that the group members can take with them that reminds them of the group and their participation in the group.

Equipment/Materials Needed: Writing utensil and paper, one for each member of the group. The facilitator could precut the paper into shapes, such as a heart or star, to add extra symbolic imagery. The facilitator should have a paper as well.

Age/Gender/Cultural Considerations: Appropriate for children about 8 years of age and up; appropriate for any gender.

Framing Questions: What makes our group special? What have we learned from each other? What have we learned about each other? What do we value in each other?

Directions for Activity:

1. Instruct each group member to get a paper and a pencil/pen/marker.
2. On the top corner of the paper, each member writes their name.
3. Ask each group member to pass their paper to the person sitting to their right. Then ask: What do you value about this person? What makes them a special group member?
4. They can write their answer anonymously or sign it.
5. Each person will have one minute to think of and write down an answer.
6. After the time is up, pass the paper in the same direction until each member has had one minute to write something on the paper for each group member.
7. The paper should eventually end up back in the original person's hands after completing a full circle around the group.
8. When the paper comes back to the original owner, they can take a moment to read the comments.

Clinical Segues and Questions:
What did it feel like to think of something positive for each group member?
How did you react to reading something positive about yourself?
How does it feel to know what others value in you?
How will you remember this group?
How will you remember your contributions to this group?
For Whom Would This Activity Be Appropriate, and for Whom Would It Not Be Appropriate?

This activity creates a lovely memory of the group. However, if there is a disgruntled or out of sync member of the group, it would be very destructive for them to write mean or cruel things about the other group members. If you believe that the group has really congealed, this is a powerful closer. If you think a group member cannot be trusted to behave appropriately, then use tap-a-roo (described in Chapter 11) as a closer instead.

Youth

Adolescents developmentally are trying to figure out who they are and who they are not, what is important to them, who is important to them, what they want to do with their lives, and what kind of adult they want to be. Youth take more risks than children or adults and tend to be more impulsive; thus for many, being active is more comfortable for them.

They are also keenly aware of other youth and how others relate to them as well. They often contemplate impressions that they are sending outward and receiving from other youth. Thus, clinical groups can be invaluable for youth as a place to be heard, valued, and understood.

Additionally, the plasticity of the brain through adolescence is an important and positive fact for clinicians, in that adolescent brains are not yet fully formed, and with the proper nurturance and stimulation, growth is still possible. Additionally, therapeutic techniques which support the full body and full mind and stimulate connections between hemispheres of the brain are particularly effective for youthful clients experiencing trauma (Uhernik, 2017). Therefore, Experiential Therapy is a very effective modality with youth.

Helium Hoop/Helium Pole

Time Duration: 10–20 minutes

Purpose/Objective: For a group to be given a simple task that becomes far more challenging than they thought

Age/Gender/Cultural Considerations: All ages, all genders

Equipment Needed: A hula hoop or a length of PVC pipe

Risk Assessment: Ensure that every member of the group is physically able to slowly maneuver to the ground and then back up again.

Framing Question: I filled this hoop/pole with helium. Can you as a group defy gravity and move it from shoulder height to the ground and back to shoulder height again, while holding it on your fingertip?

Directions for Activity:

1. Everyone places one finger on the underside of the hoop/pole.
2. Group members cannot "hook" the hula hoop or pole; they must have a straight finger.
3. Each group member needs to have contact with the hoop/pole all the time with their finger.
4. If any group member loses contact with the hoop/pole, the hoop/pole needs to return back to the initial starting position at shoulder height and the group needs to begin again.
5. As a group, they need to lower the hoop to the ground and then raise it back to shoulder height.

Clinical Segues and Questions:

Who thought this would be easy?

What do you do when something you thought would take five minutes takes much longer?

Were you more or less patient that you thought?

Did you want to give up?

How many of you wanted to blame someone else in the group?

What was your stress level?

Was conflict resolution needed?

Was problem-solving used?

Was there group leadership?

What was your level of frustration?

For Whom Would This Activity Be Appropriate, and for Whom Would It Not Be Appropriate?

This activity is suitable for any age, gender, and ability. It may be harder for individuals with low frustration tolerance. Additionally, if they become more frustrated, they will be worse and worse at the activity. The activity may need to be paused to have a moment to refocus before beginning the group again.

M&M Game

Time Duration: 15–30 minutes

Purpose/Objective: The purpose of this activity is to allow group members to recognize individual differences and commonalities in the group, and learn something new about fellow group members.

Age/Gender/Cultural Considerations: This activity is modifiable based on age, environment, and level of group comfort. The questions associated with M&M colors can be modified based on the development of the group members as well as the group subject matter. It is appropriate for any gender.

Equipment/Materials Needed: Individual size M&M bags or any other multicolor candy

Risk Assessment: Minimal risk, potential risk due to self-disclosure or activating due to question topics

Framing Questions: How do we learn new things about each other, and how are these things relatable to ourselves?

Directions for Activity:

1. Group members sit in a circle.
2. Each group member receives an individual bag of candy and pours the contents into their hand or a napkin to see the different colors, without eating the candy.
3. The facilitator asks them to first see how many blue M&Ms they have.
4. Then the facilitator states: for each blue M&M. think about a superpower you would like to have.
5. Then everyone goes around the circle naming the superpower(s) they would like to have. They are able to name the number of superpowers by the number of blue M&Ms they have. If they have no blue M&Ms, they can still state one superpower to the group. After they have stated their superpowers, they can eat their blue M&Ms.
6. Then the same procedure happens for the red M&Ms, green M&Ms, and so forth, until each color of M&M has been discussed.
7. You can attach any question to the color of the M&M, depending on the focus of the group. For instance, you could use:

Blue: If you were a superhero what would your power be?
Red: When was a time that you felt proud of yourself?
Yellow: What will success look like for you?
Green: What motivates you to do your best work?
Brown: What would you like to learn to do in the future?
Orange: Who do you admire?
Clinical Segues and Questions:
Did you learn new information about group members?
Did you realize you have more similarities to other group members than you thought?
Did it feel comfortable or uncomfortable to share personal information with the group?

Did you have difficulties with any of the questions? Why?

For Whom Would This Activity Be Appropriate, and for Whom Would It Not Be Appropriate?

This activity can be played with all age groups. The questions can be modified to fit the needs of the group. Be careful not to use peanut M&Ms due to allergies. With eating-disordered clients the actual eating of the M&Ms may be difficult for them. They do not have to eat the M&Ms.

Stuck on You

Time Duration: 15–30 minutes

Purpose/Objective: Let group members know how they are appreciated

Age/Gender/Cultural Considerations: This can be done with any age group or gender as long as they can read and write.

Equipment/Materials Needed: Sticky notes and writing utensils

Risk Assessment: Minimal risk. This can be done as a closer, like pass the paper. If you think that a group member cannot write positive notes of appreciation on the sticky notes, it is better to use tap-a-roo (described in Chapter 11).

Framing Question: How do we let our group members know that we appreciate them?

Directions for Activity:

1. The facilitator gives each group member a writing utensil and the same number of sticky notes as members in the group.
2. Every group member writes one thing that they appreciate about each group member on a sticky note. Make sure they write the group member's name on the top of the sticky note.
3. Once everyone has finished writing the sticky notes, then they stick the notes on each person's back.
4. When everyone is done, the facilitator takes the notes off each person's back and reads them aloud to the group and then hands them to the person who had them on their back.

Clinical Segues and Questions:

How was it to write how you appreciate your group members?

How did the notes make you feel when they were read out loud?

Were you surprised by some of the things that were said?

Did you know you had such a positive influence on others?

For Whom Would This Activity Be Appropriate, and for Whom Would It Not Be Appropriate?

This activity is suitable for any age, gender. It engenders a lot of positive feelings with the group and makes them feel connected and appreciated by group members. However, if you have a cantankerous or hostile group member, it would be devastating to hear mean or spiteful things, so if there is any possibility that they will not write appropriate appreciations then the activity should be avoided.

Couples

In Sternberg's seminal triangular theory of love (1986), he proposes that enduring complete love between adults needs to have three components: passion, intimacy, and commitment. He defines passion as "the drives that lead to romance, physical attraction, and sexual consummation" (Sternberg, 1986, p. 119). Intimacy is defined as "feelings of closeness, connectedness, and bondedness in loving relationships" (Sternberg, 1986, p. 119), and commitment is defined as "the decision that one loves another and the commitment to maintain that love" (p. 119). If one of the components is weak or nonexistent, the relationship is not functioning optimally. Experiential Therapy is an excellent therapeutic intervention to support the fully functioning triadic components of love in the couple dyad.

Experiential Therapy enlists the whole of each individual and challenges the couple to see their relationship in a more holistic and more positive light. Often in couples therapy the partners have become so entrenched in their own "camps" that they no longer laugh or play with each other. Experiential Therapy helps the couple remember what they liked about each other and why they fell in love with each other in the first place. Once the spark is rekindled, the relationship can grow again.

Sit to Stand

Time Duration: 10 minutes

Purpose/Objective: To practice trusting each other through cooperation

Age/Gender/Cultural Considerations: Appropriate for children about 8 years of age and up. Appropriate for any gender. Some religions forbid touch between male and females in public.

Equipment/Materials Needed: None

Risk Assessment: Minimal risk. If the couple is unable or unwilling to sit on the floor it will be impossible to do.

Framing Question: How can we support each other to be successful in getting up?

Directions for Activity:

1. With your partner, sit on the ground back-to-back.
2. Slowly try to stand up.
3. Lean on each other for support.
4. First try to get up by linking arms.
5. Then do it again a second time, with only touching each other's back to get up.
6. Then try it a third time in silence.

Clinical Segues and Questions:

Was this easy or difficult?

How did it feel to lean into your partner?

What made you more or less successful in each round of the activity?

What made you feel like a team?

When were there other times your partner helped you get up?

Did you let your partner know you appreciated the help to get up?

How can you help your partner to get "up" in the future?

For Whom Would This Activity Be Appropriate, and for Whom Would It Not Be Appropriate?

This works well with most couples. Couples with height or weight disparities can make this activity work, they just need to be more patient.

Face to Face or Back to Back

Time Duration: Approximately 10 minutes

Purpose/Objective: How do we see each other, and how do we support each other?

Age/Gender/Cultural Considerations: Appropriate for children about 8 years of age and up; appropriate for any gender. Some religions forbid touch between male and females in public. Some cultures find eye contact disrespectful.

Equipment/Materials Needed: None.

Risk Assessment: Minimal risk.

Framing Question: Do we use our eyes to see each other and our hands to support each other?

Directions for Activity:

1. Partners should sit comfortably facing each other, close enough that their knees are touching or almost touching.
2. Partners need to look into each other's eyes. They need to continue to gaze upon each other until you tell them to stop (approximately 2–3 minutes).
3. When the 2–3 minutes are over, have one partner turn their back to the other partner.
4. Direct the partner facing the other's back to gently place their hands directly on their partner's back, behind their heart.
5. The partner with their back turned should lean back into their partner's hands. The partners can have their eyes open or shut.
6. Remain in this position for approximately 2–3 minutes.
7. Before the time is over, have the person with the hand on the partner's back send a silent message to their partner. (Have them share with each other during the clinical segues what their message was.)
8. Have partners switch positions and repeat.

Clinical Segues and Questions:

How was it to look at each other for that long?

Did you see anything that you had not noticed before or had forgotten about each other?

Was it comfortable or uncomfortable to look at each other for so long? Why do you think so? Did this evoke any other strong emotions or feelings?

How was it to look at their back?

Did you prefer to be supported by or supporting your partner?

How does this align with how you usually feel in the relationship?

What was the message you sent to your partner?

For Whom Would This Activity Be Appropriate, and for Whom Would It Not Be Appropriate?

This works with most couples. If couples are very angry with each other, looking at each other can be difficult; thus you may want to reverse the order and do the touching of the partner's back first.

Mine Field

Time Duration: 20–30 minutes

Purpose/Objective: To understand better how to effectively communicate and be heard

Age/Gender/Cultural Considerations: This activity is appropriate for all ages, 8 and up. It works for various group sizes (minimum of two participants). Activity can be modified for skill level. It is appropriate for any gender.

Equipment/Materials Needed: "Mines" can be paper/plastic plates, beanbags, cones, foam noodles, and so on. The mines are any objects that can be used to block the partner's path. DO NOT use objects made of hard materials (e.g., rocks or metal). Blindfolds or bandanas are also needed.

Risk Assessment: Minimal physical risk. Participants will be blindfolded or asked to keep eyes closed; remember, it is always challenge by choice. The individual's comfort level in not using sight should be considered. Be cautious of blindfolding as it can provoke trust issues or activate post-traumatic reactions. Be sure the area that is the "minefield" is free from hazardous objects and is a flat area of ground. This activity should not be done early in therapy. If they have completed military service in a war area using mines or they are a refugee/immigrant from an area where mines were used, this could be very activating and should not be used.

Framing Question: How can we give directions so that we are understood?

Directions for Activity:

1. Choose an appropriate area.
2. Distribute the "mines" across the minefield.
3. Explain that the goal is for the blindfolded (closed-eyed) person to walk from one side of the minefield to the other, avoiding the "mines" by listening to the verbal instructions of their partner.
4. Allow the pair a short period of planning time to decide on their verbal commands and then begin the activity.
5. If a partner runs into a "mine," they must return to the beginning of the minefield.
6. When they make it through the minefield, have partners swap roles to return through the minefield again.

Clinical Segues and Questions:
What was frustrating?
What was helpful?
Did you trust your partner?
Did you trust yourself?
What did your partner do or say to help you feel safe and secure?
What could your partner have done to help make you feel safer and more secure?
What communication strategies worked best?
Did you learn anything about how you can better communicate effectively?

What were the consequences of not trusting your partner?

What were the consequences of not paying attention to your partner?

Was it easier to be blindfolded (eyes closed) and follow instructions or to give instructions?

Why do you think this is so?

Is this like other spheres of your life?

With Whom Would This Work Well, and With Whom Would It Not Work Well?

It works well with most couples. However, if they are really not listening to each other, it will highlight these issues and cause the activity to fail. This is not necessarily negative; it just means that therapy really needs to focus on communication and speaking to be understood and not just heard.

Experiential Therapy Activities in Nature for Couples

As stated in Chapter 8, "Experiential Therapy in the Natural Realm," there are a multitude of outdoor activities that can be done throughout the year. Having a couple take part in an outdoor activity together helps them spend time in nature reconnecting with each other.

On the day of the event, it is extremely important to reiterate the philosophy of "challenge by choice" to the couple before beginning the Experiential Therapy activity in nature. Additionally, each partner, before beginning, should articulate their personal and couple goal for the activity and the day. Help partners remember the goals of their partner. This helps ensure that they support and encourage each other throughout the day, as well as not pushing them past the goal they have set. Because many outdoor activities take a considerable amount of time, as well as energy, the full effect of the activity may take days to be fully comprehended by the couple. Clinical segues after the activity always occur, but they should also occur at the beginning of the next session when you see the couple again. Some couples will not be able to fully appreciate the Experiential Therapy activity in nature until they have returned to their everyday existence and have processed the experience.

Often new confidence in their relationship is found while experiencing nature, which carries over to the other spheres of their lives. Outdoor Experiential Therapy activities have a way of waking up a couple so that they can fully appreciate, value, and enjoy each other again. It can also increase the couple's tenacity and willingness to persevere when obstacles or disappointments occur in their lives and gives them opportunities to see their partner with new or renewed appreciation. Experiential Therapy supports the couple to move out from their comfort zone and challenges each partner to embrace an increased vitality in their relationship.

Families

Families function as a system. Change in one member of the family ripples through the system, affecting all the other members, as well as the overall stability of the family. It is a delicate balance between change and stability. Conceptually, "[a] family is not just a collection of individual family members, but a whole that is greater than the sum of its parts" (2019, p. 1). Individual family member's behaviors and actions are understood within the context of the family system. In Family Systems Therapy (FST) the clinician joins the family to create change within the family (Laser-Maira et al., 2019). The clinician creates an atmosphere in the sessions in which family members talk to each other and not just to the clinician. The clinician listens to what the family is saying and hears the distinct and different family voices and sees how they fit or do not fit together to tell the family story.

Using Experiential Therapy allows the clinician to better see how the family functions in a more natural environment than the confines of the clinical office. It is an amazing opportunity not only for assessment, but also to intervene in real time while they are interacting with each other and to have meaningful clinical segues where all family members are heard and validated.

Tarp Flip/Magic Carpet Ride

Time Duration: 10–20 minutes

Purpose/Objective: To problem-solve collectively and to effectively communicate

Age/Gender/Cultural Considerations: Can be used with all ages and genders

Equipment/Materials Needed: A tarp, blanket, or rug

Risk Assessment: Low risk, though family members will be in very close proximity to each other, which could be activating.

Framing Question: How do we flip the tarp/carpet /rug over and not lose anyone in the process?

Directions for Activity:

1. A tarp/carpet/rug is laid on the ground that is big enough for all family members to stand on.
2. All family members stand on the tarp/carpet/rug.

3. Family members must flip the tarp/carpet/rug over completely without anyone touching the ground outside of the carpet with their hand or foot.

4. If someone touches the ground, they must start over from the beginning.

Clinical Segues and Questions:

Did all family members contribute to solutions to flip the tarp/carpet/rug?

Were all family members heard?

Did you feel like your ideas were heard?

Did you have to try lots of different strategies?

Do you feel like you worked collectively?

Did you feel there was conflict during the activity?

How did it feel to be so physically close to each other?

Did you feel like all family members had a role?

Were all family members heard?

Was this easier or harder than you were expected?

For Whom Would This Activity Be Appropriate, and for Whom Would It Not Be Appropriate?

It may be inappropriate for some physical disabilities with mobility issues. It may be activating and thus inappropriate for individuals who have physical or sexual trauma due to having to be close to other family members. This activity may be challenging for groups who generally struggle with touching or being close to each other. It can be modified by using a larger tarp/carpet/rug.

Marble Run

Time Duration: 20 minutes

Purpose/Objective: To better communicate with each other and to problem-solve

Age/Gender/Cultural Considerations: This activity works well for children aged 6 and older and all genders. All family members will need to be mobile and have the ability to move quickly.

Equipment/Materials Needed: 10–30 marbles, a container, one piece of PVC tubing, cut in half lengthwise, 8″–12″ long, per family member

Risk Assessment: The risk is low; however, because family members are moving quickly, they should be aware of their surroundings and wear shoes that they can run in.

Framing Question: How many marbles can we move to the other side of the field and place in the container using just the PVC pipes?

Directions for Activity:

1. Family members line up in a straight line before the starting line.
2. Place a container 20 to 30 feet from the starting line.
3. Each family member is given a piece of PVC pipe.
4. Explain to family members that they have to use the PVC pipe as a chute for the marbles to roll through.
5. Each family member's PVC pipe needs to touch the next family members PVC pipe so that the marble will roll from one PVC pipe to the next.
6. The family members cannot use their fingers or any other part of their body to touch or to change the speed or the direction of the marble.
7. The family members need to take turns so that each family member in their turn uses their PVC pipe to have the marble roll.
8. Family members must stay in a straight line unless they are moving to the front of the line after the marble has rolled through their PVC pipe.
9. When the marble is on their PVC pipe, family members cannot move their feet.
10. If a marble falls, the family must begin again at the starting line.
11. Once they have successfully gotten the marble into the container at the other end, they can run back to the starting line to move another marble to the container.
12. Set your timer for 20 minutes; at the end of the 20 minutes, stop the activity and see how many marbles ended up in the container.

Clinical Segues and Questions:

Did all family members contribute to find solutions to move the marble down to the container?

Were all family members heard?

Did you feel like your ideas were heard?

Did you have to try lots of different strategies?

Do you feel like you worked collectively?

Did you feel there was conflict during the activity?

Did you feel like all family members had a role?

Were all family members heard?

Was this easier or harder than you expected?

How did you communicate during the activity?

What was the most challenging aspect of the activity?

Was it frustrating when someone else dropped a marble?

How did it feel when you dropped a marble?

For Whom Would This Activity Be Appropriate, and for Whom Would It Not Be Appropriate?

The activity would not work well with individuals with physical impairments who cannot move quickly or those with visual impairments. There is some frustration in the activity, so the facilitator should monitor the family member's frustration tolerance.

Skittles Game

Time Duration: 15–30 minutes
Purpose/Objective: The purpose of this activity is to allow family members to be heard.

Age/Gender/Cultural Considerations: This activity is effective for those age 6 and older and for all genders.

Equipment/Materials Needed: Individual size Skittles bags or any other multicolor candy

Risk Assessment: Minimal risk, potential risk due to self-disclosure or activating due to question topic

Framing Questions: How do we listen, learn, and appreciate our family members?
Directions for Activity:

1. Family members sit in a circle.
2. Each family member receives an individual bag of candy and pours the contents into their hand or a napkin to see the different colors, without eating the candy.
3. The facilitator asks them to first see how many green skittles they have.
4. Then facilitator states, for each green skittle family members need to state a word that they would use to describe themselves.
5. Then everyone goes around the circle naming a word(s) that they would use to describe themselves. They are able to name the number of words by the number of green skittles they have. If they have no green skittles, they can still state one word to describe themselves. After they have stated their words, they can eat their green skittles.
6. Then the same procedure happens for the purple, orange, and so forth, until each color of skittle has been discussed.
7. You can attach any question to the color of the skittles, depending on the focus of the session. For instance, you could use:

Green: Words to describe yourself
Purple: Things you'd like to change/improve about yourself
Orange: Things you'd like to change/improve about your family
Red: Things you worry about
Yellow: Good things about your family.

Clinical Segues and Questions:

Did you learn new information about family members?

Were you aware of your family member's thoughts?

Did you realize you have more similarities to other family members than you thought?

Did it feel comfortable or uncomfortable to share personal information with family members?

Did you have difficulties with any of the questions? Why?

For Whom Would This Activity Be Appropriate, and for Whom Would It Not Be Appropriate?

This activity can be played with most families. The questions can be modified to fit the needs of the family and what they are experiencing. With eating-disordered clients the actual eating of the candy may be difficult; thus they do not have to eat the candy. This activity is obviously similar to the M&M game. We have found that a little treat during an Experiential Therapy session frequently supports the process of therapy for both children and adults.

Next Chapter

In the next chapter, we will discuss some particular clinical groups that have benefited from Experiential Therapy so that you can understand the versatility of this modality.

Chapter 11
Experiential Therapy Activities With Specific Group Characteristics

We want to share with you some particular groups for which we use Experiential Therapy. These may not be the specific populations that you work with, but you can see how versatile Experiential Therapy is for a variety of populations. This also gives you more activities that you can modify for your own particular clientele. The groups that we see in our practice are: human trafficking survivors, veterans and military service members, individuals with substance use disorders (SUDs), juvenile justice–involved youth, and grief groups. We have found Experiential Therapy beneficial to this wide array of clientele.

Survivors of Human Trafficking

Human trafficking is a clandestine activity in which domestic and foreign nationals, through force, fraud, or coercion, have their labor, including sex, exploited (Laser-Maira et al., 2018). The vulnerability and lack of power or influence these survivors often feel make the road to recovery slow and difficult (Laser-Maira et al., 2016). Sadly, those who have experienced prior abuse are more likely to have multiple victimizations (Barnes et al., 2009; Finkelhor et al., 2009; Finkelhor et al., 2007; Finkelhor et al., 2005; Lahav & Elklit, 2016; Laser et al., 2019). For instance, an individual who has been sex trafficked very likely was previously sexually abused (Laser-Maira, Peach, et al., 2019); thus clinical therapy needs to not only work through the current events, but also attend to the earlier events (Laser-Maira et al., 2020). Additionally, if the traumatic experience is committed by a trusted individual (e.g., domestic violence/interpersonal violence) or caretaker (e.g., physical abuse or sexual abuse), the effects of the trauma are felt more profoundly (American Psychiatric Association, 2013). Sadly, in human trafficking a trusted individual is often the person who manipulates, grooms, or offers a better life to these unsuspecting victims to entice them into the "life." Thus, establishing trust and rapport takes time. We have found that Experiential

Understanding and Effectively Utilizing Experiential Therapy. Julie Anne Laser and Nicole Nicotera,
Oxford University Press. © Oxford University Press (2025). DOI: 10.1093/9780197757581.003.0011

Therapy is very effective with this population since they are unpacking so many issues from their past victimization, and movement and being outdoors is very therapeutic.

Loving Kindness Meditation

Time Duration: About 15 minutes

Purpose/Objective: Loving Kindness meditation is a well-known and used meditation practice to develop the mental habit of sending positive feelings out to the world and receiving them as well. We have modified it to only include sending out positive feelings to oneself and sending out and receiving positive sentiments only to people they identify as a friend or loved one.

Age/Gender/Cultural Considerations: All ages and genders

Equipment/Materials Needed: An open mind

Risk Assessment: Low risk unless personally having a very hard time

Framing Question: Consider the words that I will state. Let them wash over you. Consider how they make you feel. Consider how you are breathing, your heart rate, and your level of comfortability. As we repeat this more times, does this change?

Directions for Activity:

1. Have individuals find a comfortable sitting position, either with their eyes closed or gazing down.
2. Take a moment to become centered and present.
3. Then the facilitator has the group members consider these words, which they can repeat to themselves quietly or out loud:
   May I be filled with loving kindness.
   May I be held in loving kindness.
   May I feel connected and calm.
   May I accept myself just as I am.
   May I be happy.
   May I know the natural joy of being alive.
4. Now think of a **loved one** to center your thoughts on. We will again repeat the mantra.
   May you be filled with loving kindness.
   May you be held in loving kindness.
   May you feel my love now. May you accept yourself just as you are.
   May you be happy.
   May you know the natural joy of being alive.

5. Now think about your awareness moving out from you in all directions. May all beings be filled with loving kindness. May all beings be happy. May all beings awaken and be free. May all beings be happy.

6. Take a moment to open your eyes again and rejoin the group.

Clinical Segues and Questions:

Ask for general comments and reactions.

How did it feel to express love for yourself?

Is this hard or easy?

How did it feel to express love for loved ones?

How did it feel to express love everywhere?

What insights into yourself does that give you?

What came up for you emotionally? Physically?

Did you connect it to other spheres in your life?

Did this give you comfort or pain, or both?

Do you think this is something you could do daily? Weekly? Ever again?

For Whom Would This Activity Be Appropriate, and for Whom Would It Not Be Appropriate? Immature groups or untrusting groups may not want to share.

Bull in China Shop

Time Duration: 20–40 minutes

Purpose/Objective: Problem-solving activity needing group cohesion

Age/Gender/Cultural Considerations: School age and up can do the activity; a minimum of three participants is needed; any gender.

Equipment/Materials Needed: A 3–4-inch ring, a ball that can balance on that ring, an 8-foot length of rope per group member. Tie the end of each rope around the ring. A bucket placed at the end is also needed.

Risk Assessment: Minimal risk. There is some frustration, however. The ropes should not be wrapped around hands to avoid rope burns.

Framing Question: How do we transport the ball so that it does not fall?

Directions for Activity:

1. We are pretending that the ball balancing on the ring is very fragile and should be carefully transported to the bucket.
2. Each person needs to hold on to the end of one of the ropes.

3. The group needs to carefully transport the ball to the basket.
4. The basket is placed at a distance from where they start.
5. If the ball drops, the group members will need to go back to where they began and move the ball to the basket again.

Clinical Segues and Questions:

What skills did the group need to use in order to transport the ball?

Did the group use these skills well? Why or why not?

How did you communicate?

Who were the leaders of the group?

Were the leaders helpful?

Did the leaders remain the same or were they fluid?

Did you think of a solution to transport the ball before others did?

Did you or did you not share your solution with the group?

How do you get your ideas heard?

Was your group open to hearing a variety of different plans and ideas?

How was it to be a group member?

What skills do you need to create a plan and execute a plan?

How did it feel to start over from the beginning?

Did motivation increase or decrease when you had to start over?

How does this apply to achieving goals in your life?

How does it feel to start over many times in life?

How do you stay strong?

How do you become more resilient?

For Whom Would This Activity Be Appropriate, and for Whom Would It Not Be Appropriate?

Group members who have a hard time being part of a team or have a low frustration tolerance will have a more difficult time with the activity.

The Logos Approach

Additionally, we want to highlight the Experiential Therapy in nature work that is specifically being done by Logos with human trafficking survivors. Logos Healing Institute, founded by Chelsea Van Essen and Jessica Roberts in 2018, was created to provide access to wilderness spaces with clinical trauma therapy for human trafficking survivors, a population that historically has had little access to wilderness spaces. Since its inception, Logos has focused on providing evidence-based, complex trauma-specific clinical therapy services to adult survivors of human trafficking. Logos provides these services in a group-intensive format that takes place in backcountry wilderness environments.

Logos provides the necessary outdoor equipment for each human trafficking survivor and operates with a base-camp model. This includes a kitchen/communal area, a group programming tent, and individual participant tents. The intensive sessions last five days. Each morning begins with a mindfulness practice, including a body-based movement practice. This is followed by a morning group therapy session, an Experiential Therapy in nature session (either hiking, summit attempt, or rock climbing), unprogrammed free time, and afternoon Experiential Therapy activities. It is an opportunity for survivors to both grow in nature and grow in their resilience. It has been extremely successful in helping survivors make important gains in their well-being and resilience.

Veterans and Military Service Members

Active-duty service members and veterans who have seen the horrors of war sometimes come home as changed people. They often find it difficult to articulate their experiences, feelings, and thoughts associated with those experiences to others in their life. Active-duty service members and veterans are often in need of clinical therapy to make sense of the things they have witnessed and experienced when they were in the war zone (Laser & Stephens, 2011). But many are less inclined to seek out traditional talk therapy. We have found that Experiential Therapy is a very effective modality with this population. The combination of being active and outdoors helps to support their resilience, growth, and well-being.

Win/Win

Time Duration: 10 minutes

Purpose/Objective: To demonstrate how fighting over the same goal limits the positive outcomes

Age/Gender/Cultural Considerations: Appropriate for all ages and genders. Consider possible food allergies when purchasing the candy (e.g., soy, dairy, or tree nut allergies).

Equipment Needed: Bag of small candies (e.g., Skittles, M&Ms, jellybeans). Avoid Reese's pieces or Peanut M&Ms due to possible nut allergies.

Risk Assessment: Minimal risk as this activity can be done sitting down. It may be impor-tant to express overtly that it is not okay to be overly aggressive at winning so as to injure their partner's fingers, hand, or wrist.

Framing Activity: How many times can you pin your partner's thumb in 30 seconds? For every pinning of your partner's thumb, you will win a piece of candy.

Directions for Activity:

1. Use standard "thumb wars" rules: Need to use one's thumb while holding the hand of one's partner to pin the partner's thumb down. The arm or the wrist cannot be moved to gain control over the other person's thumb.
2. Round 1: Let them know 30 seconds on timer, go.
3. After the first round, distribute the candies according to how many times each partner won. If one partner won 3 times in 30 seconds, that person gets 3 candies, and if the other partner won 2 times, that person get 2 candies, and so on.
4. Round 2: Let them know 30 seconds on timer, go.
5. After the second round, distribute the candies according to how many times each partner won. If one partner won 3 times in 30 seconds, that person gets 3 candies, and if the other partner won 4 times, they get 4 candies, and so on.
6. Discuss if there were any changes in how many candies each won in the second round.
7. Ask if there was one winner and one loser thus far, or they both were winners in the second round?
8. Round 3: Let them know 30 seconds on timer, go.
9. If a pair has not already determined what it takes to win a lot of candies, secretly tell just one partner the secret to winning: Each partner lets the other win over and over.
10. After the third round, distribute the candies according to how many times each partner won. If one partner won 30 times in 30 seconds, that person gets 30 candies, and if the other partner won 30 times, they get 30 candies, and so on.
11. Discuss if there were any changes in how many candies each won in the third round.
12. Ask if there was one winner and one loser, or were they both were winners in the third round?

Clinical Segues and Questions:
What did it feel like when you won?

What did it feel like to lose?

What did it take to win big?

How did your feelings change toward your partner when you learned how to win big?

Can we both be winners?

Is it okay to let others win sometimes?

How can you use this activity in other aspects of your life?

Do we have to win all the time to feel okay about ourselves?

For Whom Would This Activity Be Appropriate, and for Whom Would It Not Be Appropriate?

For some, they may feel that the way to win is to "cheat" and they may feel angry with the activity. Unpack that and talk through why they feel that they have to compete to win. This activity often brings forth a long discussion about core values: of winning, losing, competing, following rules, taking turns, and sharing.

Ask for Help

Time Duration: 20–40+ minutes

Purpose/Objective: To experience the emotions that comes with an inability to solve a problem

Age/Gender/Cultural Considerations: All ages above 6, all genders, need to be able to walk

Equipment/Materials Needed: Long rope(s) and blindfolds/bandanas for each group member

Risk Assessment: Emotional safety issues with blindfolds need to be considered; emotional safety of feeling foolish, embarrassed, or frustrated.

Framing Question: This is an activity that is meant to induce strong feelings. Remember you can always ask for help. When you feel frustrated, can you ask for help?

Directions for Activity Stated to Participants:

1. The goal is to get yourself out of the maze.
2. You will enter the maze one by one, blindfolded (or eyes closed if they do not want to wear a blindfold).
3. Once you are in the maze, you cannot untie any knots in the rope.
4. Once you are in the maze, there is no talking allowed.
5. Once you are in the maze, you must walk slowly, one hand on the rope and one hand out in front of you to not run into others in the maze.

6. Once you are in the maze, raise your hand if you need help.
7. Remember that you can always ask for help and help will be given!

Directions for Activity Not Stated to Participants:

1. You should have a co-facilitator for this activity.
2. One facilitator stays in the center of the "maze" to monitor the group members in the "maze."
3. The other facilitator brings group members, one by one, blindfolded (or eyes closed) into the "maze."
4. Make sure the "maze" is not visible to the group.
5. The "maze" in actuality is a circle.
6. When group members are brought into the "maze" by the one facilitator, they should walk slowly, and the facilitator should place them away from the others on the circle.
7. Every two to three minutes, the facilitator in the maze should say, "Remember you can always ask for help and help will be given!"
8. When a group member asks for help, the facilitator in the center of the "maze" comes over, and states, "Remember you can always ask for help and help will be given!" and gently removes their blindfold/bandana and reminds them again that there is no talking in the maze or near the maze.
9. The group members who have "found their way out of the maze" by asking for help are asked to sit quietly outside of the maze until all group members have found their way out of the maze.
10. If there are two or fewer group members in the "maze" and they have been circling for over 25 minutes, the facilitator in the "maze" should let the group members know that the maze will be closed in 5 minutes and then add again, "Remember you can always ask for help and help will be given!"
11. Once the last group members ask for help or the time is up, the activity is over.

Clinical Segues and Questions:
What feelings did this bring up in you?
Did you wish you would have waited to ask for help?
Did you wish you would have asked sooner?
What narratives did you tell yourself in your head before you decided to ask for help?
What did you tell yourself in order to allow yourself to ask for help?
If you did not ask for help, what narratives prevented you from asking for help?
Do you ask for help in your real life?
Whom can you ask to help you in your real life?
Why is it so hard to ask for help?

For Whom Would This Activity Be Appropriate, and for Whom Would It Not Be Appropriate?

This works well for most people. It usually ends with a long discussion of how hard it is to ask for help, their fears of asking for help, and what they lose and gain by asking for help. It is often a breakthrough session for military folk, but it is also a profound experience for most clients. Some years later, some still talk about the "ask for help" activity in sessions.

Substance Use Disorders

Substance use disorders (SUDs) are defined as the recurrent use of drugs or alcohol that causes significant impairment to health and mental health functioning, and failure to meet responsibilities at home, work, or school (SAMHSA, 2019). Many individuals with trauma histories may use substances to numb the pain or block thinking about the traumatic event (Laser-Maira, Blair, et al., 2019). Instead of getting the help that they need for the trauma, they use substances instead (Laser & Wallis, 2014). Individuals who are experiencing chronic pain often use substances to reduce their physical pain. This may be the root cause in cannabis use disorders and opioid use disorders and should be inquired about (Laser-Maira, Blair, et al., 2019). Experiential Therapy can be very useful for clients with SUDs to better understand their issues and cravings that support their SUD and to choose other options to support their sobriety.

Additionally, the client's motivation for change (Prochaska et al., 1992) needs to be assessed from: (1) no problem/nothing to change/precontemplation; (2) might change/contemplation; (3) I will change/preparation; (4) I am making a change/action; (5) I have been making changes/maintenance; (6) falling back into old patterns/relapse (CAN OCCUR ANY TIME); (7) I am competent on my own/termination. Therefore, when working with clients with SUD it is important to understand what stage of change they currently are operating in. Often family and friends will be very concerned about the client's SUD and want to intervene; however, the client may not really be in a place to work on their sobriety until they are in the preparation or action stages. We have found that being active, movement, and greater holistic engagement through Experiential Therapy is very effective with clients who are working through SUDs.

Cog in the Machine

Time Duration: 10–30 minutes
Purpose/Objective: To bring light to that we are all part of the solution

Age/Gender/Cultural Considerations: Ages 8 and older and any gender. Group members are in close proximity to each other; if this is activating a different activity should be used.

Equipment/Materials Needed: A space large enough for your group to form a chain.

Risk Assessment: Ensure that all participants' chosen motions are appropriate and respectful of others' space and identities and can be done repetitively.
Framing Questions: How does a machine work? What parts are needed?

Directions for Activity:

1. The group forms a circle.
2. The facilitator explains that for the machine to work properly, everyone needs to be part of the solution to create a machine, and for the machine to work, everyone needs to contribute their energy.
3. The group members are asked to think of a movement that they could do repeatedly to be their own "cog" in the machine.
4. The first group member goes to the center and begins their chosen motion.
5. The second participant stands near the first group member and begins their chosen motion.
6. This continues until everyone has a motion and is in line. You may need the "machine" to spiral outward from the first group member, depending on space.
7. After all group members are arranged and are completing their motions simultaneously, the facilitator will instruct the first group member to choose if they want to speed up or slow down their motion. And then ask if others want to speed up or slow down.
8. Group members should increase or decrease the speed of their motion based on the participant in front of them.

Clinical Segues and Questions:
How did it feel to be the first participant?
How did it feel to be far away from the center?
How did it feel to be close to the center?
Did you like to be part of something bigger than yourself?
How did it feel to be part of a "machine"?
What "machine parts" do you need for your sobriety?
Who makes up your machine?
What can you do to make the machine work more effectively?

Who is part of your machine for sobriety?

For Whom Would This Activity Be Appropriate, and for Whom Would It Not Be Appropriate?

This activity works well for most people; however, it would probably be advisable that the more socially anxious group members are not the early ones to be part of the machine.

Outdoor Scavenger Hunt

Time Duration: 1 hour

Purpose/Objective: Create symbols of yourself and your journey in sobriety and what you will look like living a sober life.

Age/Gender/Cultural Considerations: As long as they can move through the outdoors on their own, they can do this activity.

Equipment/Materials Needed: Cell phones *or* paper and pencils/crayons, journaling book/pad of paper, foghorn or other loud noisemaker to let the group know when time is up to return to circle.

Risk Assessment: The biggest issue is to make sure they know how far off they can wander and to make sure they can hear the noisemaker/foghorn to return. If they cannot be trusted to go very far, explain that you need to have eyes on them the entire time and rope off the area in advance where they can be.

Framing Question: How do you see yourself in nature?

Directions for Activity:

1. Explain that you are giving each of them 20 minutes of time.
2. They need to stay in the required area, and they will be called back by the loud noisemaker/ foghorn when time is up.
3. Sound the loud noisemaker/foghorn so they know what it sounds like.
4. Tell them that this is a silent activity until they come back to the group.
5. Tell them they will need to find three things.
6. First, ask them to find a tree, stone, plant, animal, natural formation that **reminds them of themselves**. If they have their cell phones, they can take a picture of it. If they don't, they can draw a picture of it with the drawing materials provided.
7. Then they need to sit and look at it for a bit and write down in their journal why the tree, stone, natural formation reminds them of themselves. What are the

characteristics of the object? Why is it important for them? Why do they see themselves that way?

8. Second, they find another tree, stone, plant, animal, natural formation that reminds them of their **journey in sobriety** and go through the same process, taking a picture of it or drawing it and then journaling about the characteristics of the object, why it is important for them, and why they see their journey in sobriety that way.

9. Then, third, you ask them to find a tree, stone, plant, animal, natural formation that is how they see themselves **living a sober life** and go through the same process, taking a picture of it or drawing it and then journaling about the characteristics of the object, why it is important for them, and why they see their living a sober life that way.

10. Tell them that when the noisemaker/ foghorn is sounded, they will come back together and share their pictures/artwork and journal entries with the group, as they choose.

Clinical Segues and Questions:

How was it to find objects in nature that represented themselves, their journey in sobriety, and living a sober life?

Was this easy or difficult?

How was it being by yourself in nature?

What did you learn about yourself doing the activity?

What did you learn about your journey in sobriety?

How do you envision your future?

How did hearing and seeing the objects that other people found affect you?

In the future, when you are feeling activated or having a tough day or having cravings, can you use these pictures of these objects in nature as support to you?

For Whom Would This Activity Be Appropriate, and for Whom Would It Not Be Appropriate?

As long as the group members have mobility (and are not runners) this will work well. Clients with more significant trauma histories sometimes do not like to be by themselves in nature very long and may want to be in closer proximity to the clinician or may return before the time is called.

Juvenile Justice–Involved Youth

We have found that many who are involved with the legal system feel particularly stigmatized by being named juvenile delinquents (Laser & Nicotera, 2021), so instead we use the term *juvenile justice–involved youth.* This connotation helps to convey their involvement with the legal system, but is less pejorative. A vast majority of youth in the juvenile justice system have a history of trauma (Laser & Nicotera, 2021).

Experiential therapy is very effective for working with youth in the juvenile justice system. The emphasis in Experiential Therapy for the body to be active and engaged while they are in clinical therapy has a very positive effect on juvenile justice–involved youth. We have found that youth in the juvenile justice system really enjoy their involvement in Experiential Therapy and make the connections from Experiential Therapy to other spheres of their life (Laser & Nicotera, 2021). Interestingly, we have found that juvenile justice–involved youth also remember the Experiential Therapy activity better than talk therapy and can access and return to the lessons learned from Experiential Therapy better than they can with talk therapy (Laser & Nicotera, 2021). We believe that their predilection for the adrenaline rush, adventure, and excitement (which may have contributed to their involvement in the juvenile justice system) naturally pairs with Experiential Therapy. Thus, Experiential Therapy is using their natural tendencies to support increased well-being and resilience.

What Do We Need and What Can Happen? ?

Time Duration: 20–30 minutes

Purpose/Objective: Clarify what we all need to be successful through the probation process and issues that can arise that are unforeseen

Age/Gender/Cultural Considerations: Need some hand-eye coordination, so the youngest age to do the activity would probably be early elementary; those who have trouble grasping with their hands may not be able to participate. Any gender can participate. Participants need to have the ability to catch and throw.

Equipment/Materials Needed: 6–8 small stuffy toys that will not hurt if they are thrown at participants.

Risk Assessment: Minimal risk in playing, some risk of disclosure in clinical segues

Framing Question: What do we all need to be successful to persevere through probation?

Directions for Activity:

1. Have the group discuss and decide on what we need/what qualities we need to possess to be successful in getting through probation.

2. Each stuffy toy represents one of those agreed-upon qualities (save 2 or more toys for later).
3. Have the group form a circle.
4. Then proceed by throwing one "quality" stuffy toy to a group member, have that group member throw to another, until everyone has been tossed the toy.
5. Then have them follow the same throwing pattern and add the second "quality" stuffy toy to throw.
6. Have them follow the pattern of throwing until all "quality" stuffy toys are tossed successfully through the circle in the same pattern.
7. Did any of them fall to the ground?
8. Do it again until the group can successfully catch and throw all of the "quality" stuffy toys through the group.
9. Then begin to discuss things that get in the way of being successful. What happens when problems happen, or our plans get changed?
10. The last two toys (or more) are named for the problems that get in the way, or can simply be named "chaos."
9. Throw the "quality" stuffy toys in the same pattern again.
10. Now, as the "quality" stuffy toys are thrown, the facilitator throws the "problem" stuffy toys to disrupt the pattern for the group.
11. Were they able to catch all the "quality" stuffy toys when the "problem" stuffy toys infiltrated the game?

Clinical Segues and Questions:

How did it feel to name the qualities you need to get through probation?
How did it feel to have success with the "quality" stuffy toys?
How did it feel when the problems entered into the circle?
Which were easier to name for you, qualities or problems?
Why do you think this was the case?
Which qualities and which problems named most resonate for you?
What happens when we have more problems thrown at us?
What makes us most vulnerable?
How can we make ourselves more resilient?
How can we stay the course through probation?
For Whom Would This Activity Be Appropriate, and for Whom Would It Not Be Appropriate?

Participants need to have the cognitive functioning to be able to think in metaphors. Participants can sit in circle if unable to stand. This activity has been very effective with juvenile justice–involved youth to articulate and remember what they need to do to make it through probation. In many groups, we would revisit and name the qualities that they decided upon at the beginning of each session.

Roses Have Thorns but Also Flowers

Time Duration: 20–30 minutes

Purpose/Objective: Each of us has parts of us that are good and parts that are less good.

Age/Gender/Cultural Considerations: Anyone who can draw, so about age 6 and above; any gender.

Equipment/Materials Needed: A piece of paper for each group member; a wide variety of markers and crayons that they can use to draw.

Risk Assessment: Minimal risk in playing, some risk of disclosure in clinical segues.

Framing Question: How do we see ourselves?

Directions for Activity:

1. Each group member should be given a piece of paper and choose the markers and crayons they want to use to draw a rose (or any flower they choose).
2. The facilitator asks them each to first draw the stem. The stem should represent the way they grew up, and they can put words along the stem.
3. The facilitator then asks them to draw the thorns of the rose on the stem, which represent the frustration, hardships, or challenges they have experienced. They can name those on each thorn if they choose.
4. Then the facilitator asks them to draw the flower, with petals that represent their successes, positive people in their life, and things they have learned.
5. If they choose, they can share their artwork.

Clinical Segues and Questions:

How did drawing the rose make you feel?

Are you surprised at how the stem looks?

Are you surprised at how many thorns are on the rose?

Are you surprised by the number of petals you have on your flower?

Did you learn anything about yourself?

How does it feel to look at your life that way?

Did you share your flower with the group?

How does sharing make you feel?

Why did you not want to share?

Don't we all have beautiful and less beautiful parts?

For Whom Would This Activity Be Appropriate, and for Whom Would It Not Be Appropriate?

This activity may not work well with individuals who have low cognitive skills or cannot use metaphors. Often the stems are very long and twisted and the rose has many thorns, but the flower itself is beautiful, and they are often very pleased by their creation.

Tap-a-Roo

Time Duration: 20–30 minutes

Purpose/Objective: This is a great closing activity.

Age/Gender/Cultural Considerations: All ages and all genders can participate.

Equipment/Materials Needed: None

Risk Assessment: There is soft physical touch of the group members' back when their eyes are closed. So, if they are bothered by touch, this needs to monitored by the facilitator for group member's activation. Facilitator must monitor to ensure all participants get appreciated. Facilitator may also participate to gently tap all participants.

Framing Question: Do we know how much we have been appreciated in our group?

Directions for Activity for Group Members:

1. Start instructing the group to get in a big circle and sit on the ground.
2. Ask one-third of the group to make a smaller circle in the middle of the circle.
3. Ask those who are sitting in the middle circle to close their eyes and put their head down.
4. Ask those who are sitting on the outer circle to stand up.
5. Explain to the outer circle standing that you will read some statements and if they feel that way about the person, they should lightly tap them on the shoulder.
6. Each statement will be read and then time will be given for the outside group to tap whomever they want in the inside group.
7. Both tappers and inside group seated members need to be completely silent.
8. They can tap as many people in the middle circle as they choose.
9. Read about 4–6 statements for people in the middle; then the second third of the group should come to the middle, and the middle people should go to the outside to tap people.
10. Read about another 4–6 statements for people in the middle, and then the third third of the group should come to the middle, and those in middle should go to the outside to tap people.
11. All the group should have an opportunity to be tapped and 2 opportunities to be a tapper.

Directions for Activity NOT Stated to Participants:

Make sure that during each statement, you (as the facilitator) go around and tap everyone on the back so that no one is neglected.

Examples of Statements: "Tap someone who . . ."

Makes you smile

You admire

Is a hard worker

You would like to be friends with

Is strong

Has a big heart

You would like to know better

Has helped you learn

Has helped you grow

Has helped you see things differently

Makes you laugh

You could cry with

You are proud of

Is amazing

Is interesting

Is fun

Is an authentic person

Is unique

Is helpful

Is kind

Is caring

Is someone you can count on

Is resilient

Is special

Is a great human being

Clinical Segues and Questions:

What did it feel like to receive these statements?

Were there any you were selected for that surprised you?

Are there any statements that you are proud of?

Was it difficult to be in the center?

What was it like to receive the statements anonymously?

Did it feel good that all the group thought these statements about you?

For Whom Would This Activity Be Appropriate, and for Whom Would It Not Be Appropriate?

This activity works well for groups who know each another. It supports a positive ending for the group.

Grief Groups

As stated in Chapter 7, David Kessler, National Grief Expert, explains, "all grief does not have trauma, But ALL trauma has grief"(personal communication, Grief Educator Training, 2023). Thus, the grief an individual may be feeling may be complicated with unexpected emotions, thoughts, and possible feelings of guilt and shame. Grief can also churn up old memories, forgotten traumas, and inequities.

There is no timeline or expiration date for grief. Everyone does grief on their own time frame, as needed. However, there are four stages of grief, from anticipatory grief before the death occurs, to acute grief when the death has just happened, to early grief in the first two years after the death, and mature grief that lasts the rest of the individual's life (Kessler, personal communication, Grief Educator Training, 2023). Therefore, at each stage of grief, the individual is most focused on different aspects of the grief. However, across all stages, the most fundamental intervention is to support the grieving individual where they are and to acknowledge the enormity of their loss (Kessler, personal communication, Grief Educator Training, 2023). Additionally, over time the clinician can help the client find meaning from the loss and honor that individual by the way they chose to move forward to fully live life again. Thus "a broken heart is also an open heart" (Kessler, personal communication, Grief Educator Training, 2023) to embrace life and living anew.

Remembrance of You

Time Duration: 15 minutes

Purpose/Objective: To hold on to a remembrance of the deceased

Age/Gender/Cultural Considerations: Appropriate for children about age 8 and up; appropriate for any gender.

Equipment/Materials Needed: Polymer clay (can be purchased at any hobby or arts and crafts store), cookie sheet, and an oven (if there is not an oven at work, you can bring this home and have it ready for the next session).

Risk Assessment: Minimal risk, though may evoke tears

Framing Question: Though your loved one is no longer with you, you will always remember them.

Directions for Activity:

1. Each group member is asked to choose three colors of clay that can represent three attributes that they appreciated about the individual. You can choose to have them share the attribute now or at the end during the clinical segues.
2. The three strands of clay are then rolled together to represent the unique cohesion of the valuable qualities that symbolized that individual.
3. After the colors have been swirled together, then the clay is formed into a disk about the size of a quarter, and a quarter-inch thick.
4. Each group member gently presses their thumb into the clay, which represents the connectedness between them.
5. The remembrance is baked in the oven, and given to each other at the next appointment as a keepsake they can have in their pocket or purse.

Clinical Segues and Questions:
What is the significance of the colors for you?
How did you translate those attributes you appreciate about your loved one into colors?
Why did you choose those attributes?
How do you react to the idea of holding on to the remembrance?
Does it help to make you feel grounded?
Does it make you feel more connected to the loved one?
Does it give you a physical remembrance that they are with you always?
For Whom Would This Activity Be Appropriate, and for Whom Would It Not Be Appropriate?

This activity works with most people. Individuals who have not allowed themselves to be creative for a long time will take longer to enter into the activity. This activity can be very sad. However, it gives each group member an opportunity to talk about their loved one. Often in other spheres of their lives, people do not ask.

Favorites Bingo

Time Duration: 20 minutes

Purpose/Objective: This is a great activity to get to know each other better in group and to learn commonalities. Often clients who are experiencing grief have had their friend circle made smaller due to prior caretaking responsibilities or losing contact with folks who have not been responsive to their needs in grief. This is an opportunity to help reduce the feelings of isolation and begin to build a community in the group again.

Age/Gender/Cultural Considerations: All ages and genders can participate.

Equipment/Materials Needed: Handout (below) copied for each group member and a writing utensil for each group member.

Risk Assessment: Low risk

Framing Question: Let's find out more about our group members.

Directions for Activity:

1. Hand out the papers and writing utensils.
2. Most will know the rules of bingo already; they need to fill in an entire row, column, or diagonal with people's information.
3. Additionally, to help them remember whom they spoke to, they should also fill in: Who: Who did you ask?, and What: What did they answer?
4. They cannot ask the same person a second question until they have asked every group member once.
5. Allow the game to go on until everyone has made a bingo.

Favorite Sport Who What	Favorite Country to Visit Who What	Favorite Food Who What	Favorite Color Who What	Favorite Dinosaur Who What
Favorite Thing to Do in Spare Time Who What	Favorite US State Who What	Favorite Hair Color Who What	Favorite Movie Who What	Favorite Animal Who What
Favorite Holiday Who What	Favorite Park to Visit Who What	Favorite Superhero Who What	Favorite Show/Series Who What	Favorite Flower Who What
Favorite Book Who What	Favorite Restaurant Who What	Favorite Junk Food Who What	Favorite Saying Who What	Favorite Pet Who What
Favorite Season Who What	Favorite Place You Have Ever Lived Who What	Favorite Dessert Who What	Favorite Song Who What	Favorite Weather Who What

Clinical Segues and Questions:

Were you surprised by your group members' answers?

Were you happy to find that you had so much in common with others?

Did some of the answers make you laugh?

Was it nice to have fun?

Was it nice to connect with others in the group?

For Whom Would This Activity Be Appropriate, and for Whom Would It Not Be Appropriate?

Most people will enjoy this activity. Even those with mobility issues can enjoy playing. Many who have been "sitting in their sad" for a while need an opportunity to laugh and enjoy themselves again. It may also bring up a discussion that laughing or being happy does not decrease the memory or the feelings for the deceased. It may spur a discussion of how they may begin to rejoin life again and how they can honor their loved one in that process.

These groups may not be the groups that you run. However, by modifying these activities they will likely work for you.

Next Chapter

In the closing chapter, we will discuss how you can evaluate Experiential Therapy's effectiveness in your organization or practice.

Chapter 12
Evaluating Experiential Therapy in Your Practice and Conclusions

We really believe that Experiential Therapy adds a great deal to one's skills as an effective clinician and helps many clients increase their well-being and resilience, especially those for whom traditional talk therapy is not a good fit. We have found that Experiential Therapy works with a wide variety of clientele, especially those who have experienced trauma.

But being researchers, as well as clinicians, we feel compelled to research its effectiveness as well. We have shared our research with you throughout the book. We would like to share the survey instruments we have created, which have been vetted by the Institutional Review Board (IRB) at our university, so you too can know not just anecdotally, but scientifically, that Experiential Therapy works in your practice. We continue to do ongoing research on Experiential Therapy so that it will become an evidenced-based practice.

We have separated the survey instruments into three different categories: (1) ongoing Experiential Therapy; (2) an eight-hour Challenge Course day with an Experiential Therapist; and (3) Logos Experiential Therapy trips with human trafficking survivors (discussed in Chapter 11).

Ongoing Experiential Therapy Evaluation

12.0 Questions Asked Week 1, 4, 8, 12 ...

1. Client number #_____;2. Session #_____ 3. Clinician(s) _____

4. Experiential Therapy Activities (all that you remember)

_____

How much do you agree with the following statements:

5. Experiential Therapy has helped me feel less alone.
1 = strongly disagree, 2 = disagree, 3 = neither agree nor disagree, 4 = agree, 5 = strongly agree

Understanding and Effectively Utilizing Experiential Therapy. Julie Anne Laser and Nicole Nicotera, Oxford University Press. © Oxford University Press (2025). DOI: 10.1093/9780197757581.003.0012

6. I have felt better emotionally since working with my clinician(s).
1 = strongly disagree, 2 = disagree, 3 = neither agree nor disagree, 4 = agree,
5 = strongly agree

7. I have gained greater self-esteem because of Experiential Therapy.
1 = strongly disagree, 2 = disagree, 3 = neither agree nor disagree, 4 = agree,
5 = strongly agree

8. My mood has improved due to Experiential Therapy.
1 = strongly disagree, 2 = disagree, 3 = neither agree nor disagree, 4 = agree,
5 = strongly agree

9. I feel less stressed due to Experiential Therapy.
1 = strongly disagree, 2 = disagree, 3 = neither agree nor disagree, 4 = agree,
5 = strongly agree

10. I have new ways to approach life situations due to Experiential Therapy.
1 = strongly disagree, 2 = disagree, 3 = neither agree nor disagree, 4 = agree,
5 = strongly agree

11. I have noticed differences in the way the people in my life respond to me because
of Experiential Therapy.
1 = strongly disagree, 2 = disagree, 3 = neither agree nor disagree, 4 = agree,
5 = strongly agree

12. I have increased my knowledge of how relationships work due to Experiential
Therapy.
1 = strongly disagree, 2 = disagree, 3 = neither agree nor disagree, 4 = agree,
5 = strongly agree

13. I have learned new skills because of Experiential Therapy.
1 = strongly disagree, 2 = disagree, 3 = neither agree nor disagree, 4 = agree,
5 = strongly agree

14. Even though I may not yet be where I want to be, my life has improved due to
Experiential Therapy.
1 = strongly disagree, 2 = disagree, 3 = neither agree nor disagree, 4 = agree,
5 = strongly agree

15. I have greater confidence in my ability to have successful relationships because of
Experiential Therapy.
1 = strongly disagree, 2 = disagree, 3 = neither agree nor disagree, 4 = agree,
5 = strongly agree

16. How hopeful do you feel about the future?
1 = not at all, 2 = a little, 3 = a fair amount, 4 = very, 5 = extremely

17. I would recommend Experiential Therapy to a friend or family member.
1 = strongly disagree, 2 = disagree, 3 = neither agree nor disagree, 4 = agree, 5 = strongly agree

Basic Demographic Information

Filled out by Clinician at the First Session Only

Client #
Gender Identity
Age
Race
Ethnicity
Level of Education
Primary language
Diagnosis (if known)

We have found that asking clients to fill out the form every 4 weeks allows them to not be overwhelmed with paperwork. It also is enough time for them to see their progress in therapy as well. If we are working with a group, couple, or a family, each group member fills out their own form.

Challenge Course Evaluation

We sometimes do a one-day eight-hour Experiential Therapy session at the Challenge Course. This is a very different day for most, and we thought we needed a particular survey to investigate the influence the day had on them. We work with Denver Parks and Recreation, which operates a high-quality facility. They have expertly trained staff who take care of the "hard skills" (equipment and its upkeep, harnesses, helmets, ropes, safety instructions, and belaying), while we do the "soft skills" of Experiential Therapy. Often the day at the Challenge Course is an extremely transformative day for the group.

12.0 Experiential Activities Evaluation (EAE)

Client _____

1. Age _____

2. What is your race/ethnicity (select all that apply)?
A. African American/Black   B. Asian   C. Hispanic/ Latino
D. Native American/Native Alaskan   E. Pacific Islander   F. White/Caucasian
G. Other_____

3. Which gender do you most identify with?
A. Female   B. Male   C. Other

4. Have you participated in a challenge course before today?   Y/N

5. If yes, number of times_____.

6. Have you participated in low elements before today?   Y/N

7. If yes, number of times_____.

8. Have you participated in high elements before today?   Y/N

9. If yes, number of times_____.

(If a question does not apply to you, do not answer.)

For the following questions, answer:

1 = disagree, 2 = somewhat disagree, 3 = neutral, 4 = agree,
5 = strongly agree

10. I believe I was fully engaged in the activities.	1	2	3	4	5
11. I thoroughly enjoyed my experience at the Challenge Course.	1	2	3	4	5
12. I thoroughly enjoyed the low elements.	1	2	3	4	5
13. I thoroughly enjoyed the high elements.	1	2	3	4	5
14. I learned something new about myself.	1	2	3	4	5
15. I grew as an individual.	1	2	3	4	5
16. I believe I'll bring these changes to my personal life beyond this experience.	1	2	3	4	5
17. I grew as a member of my group.	1	2	3	4	5
18. My experience today increased my trust of others.	1	2	3	4	5
19. My experience today increased confidence in myself.	1	2	3	4	5
20. My experience today increased my ability to make decisions.	1	2	3	4	5
21. My experience today increased my ability to problem-solve.	1	2	3	4	5
22. My experience today increased my communication with others.	1	2	3	4	5
23. I left my comfort zone.	1	2	3	4	5
24. I am glad I left my comfort zone.	1	2	3	4	5

25. Fear modified my participation in a particular activity.   1   2   3   4   5

26. I feel I am more likely to leave my comfort zone in the future.   1   2   3   4   5

27. I will be a better group member because of my experience today.   1   2   3   4   5

28. I would participate in a Challenge Course again.   1   2   3   4   5

29. I would recommend this experience to someone with similar life   1   2   3   4   5
experiences as I have.

30. I would recommend this experience to a friend/family member.   1   2   3   4   5

31. How many people do you know that could benefit from
participation in a Challenge Course? #_____

32. Comments???

Trip Evaluation

As discussed in Chapter 11, Logos Healing Institute does five-day trips with human trafficking survivors. We have been the researchers for their organization to evaluate the gains the survivors have made at the conclusion of the trip, but also the long-term residual gains that the survivors made at three months, six months, and one year after their trip. The gains have been substantial, and the long-term effect has been stable to support increased well-being and resilience in survivors. We will shortly be publishing these results.

12.0 Logos Healing Institute

Experiential Therapy Evaluation

1. #_____ 2. Date_____ 3. Age _____

4. What is your race/ethnicity (select all that apply)?
A. African American/Black   B. Asian   C. Hispanic/ Latina/o
D. Native American/Native Alaskan   E. Pacific Islander   F. White/Caucasian
G. Other_____

5. Which gender do you most identify with?
A. Female   B. Male   C. Other

6. Have you participated in experiential activities before this trip?
Y/N _____# of times

7. How long were you in "the life"? _____

8. How long have you been out of "the life"? _____

9. History of sexual abuse   Yes No

10. History of physical abuse   Yes No

11. History of emotional abuse   Yes No

12. Do you experience disassociation (check out/space out)?   Yes No

13. Have you been in clinical therapy?   Yes No

14. If yes, type of clinical therapy: _____

15. If yes, length of clinical therapy _____

For the following questions, answer:
1 = disagree, 2 = somewhat disagree, 3 = neutral, 4 = agree,
5 = strongly agree

16. I believe I was fully engaged in the experiential trip.   1   2   3   4   5

17. I thoroughly enjoyed the experiential trip   1   2   3   4   5

18. I learned something new about myself.   1   2   3   4   5

19. I feel better in my body.   1   2   3   4   5

20. I grew as an individual.   1   2   3   4   5

21. I believe I'll bring these changes to my personal life beyond this 1   2   3   4   5
experience.

22. I grew as a member of my program group.   1   2   3   4   5

23. My experience increased my trust of others.   1   2   3   4   5

24. My experience increased trust in myself.   1   2   3   4   5

25. My experience increased my confidence in decision-making.   1   2   3   4   5

26. My experience increased my ability to problem-solve.   1   2   3   4   5

27. My experience increased my communication with others.   1   2   3   4   5

28. I left my comfort zone.   1   2   3   4   5

29. I am glad I left my comfort zone.   1   2   3   4   5

30. I feel I am more likely to leave my comfort zone in the future. 1   2   3   4   5

31. I feel less alone because of the experiential trip.   1   2   3   4   5

32. I feel like I can relate to others better because of the experiential 1   2   3   4   5
trip.

33. I recognize new strengths I possess because of the experiential 1   2   3   4   5
trip.

34. I experienced the challenge by choice philosophy on the trip. 1   2   3   4   5

35. I would recommend this experience to someone with similar life 1   2   3   4   5
experiences as me.

36. I would recommend this experience to a friend/family member.   1   2   3   4   5

37. What was the most impactful part of your experience?

38. What was the least helpful part of your experience?

39. How did the wilderness/nature influence your healing on this trip?

40. Were there barriers to coming on this experiential trip? If so, what were they?

41. Other comments???

12.0 Logos Healing Institute

Experiential Therapy Evaluation, 3 Months, 6 Months, One Year Post Trip

1. #_____ 2. Date of trip_____

For the following questions answer:
1 = disagree, 2 = somewhat disagree, 3 = neutral, 4 = agree, 5 = strongly agree

3. I believe I was fully engaged in the experiential trip.   1   2   3   4   5

4. I thoroughly enjoyed the experiential trip.   1   2   3   4   5

5. I learned something new about myself.   1   2   3   4   5

6. I feel better in my body.   1   2   3   4   5

7. I grew as an individual.   1   2   3   4   5

8. I brought these changes to my personal life beyond the trip.   1   2   3   4   5

9. My experience increased my trust of others.   1   2   3   4   5

10. My experience increased trust in myself   1   2   3   4   5
11. My experience increased my confidence in decision-making.   1   2   3   4   5

12. My experience increased my ability to problem-solve.   1   2   3   4   5

13. My experience increased my communication with others.   1   2   3   4   5

14. I remind myself that I left my comfort zone.   1   2   3   4   5

15. I am glad I left my comfort zone.   1   2   3   4   5

16. I have left my comfort zone since the trip.   1   2   3   4   5

17. I feel less alone because of the experiential trip.   1   2   3   4   5

18. I feel like I can relate to others better because of the experiential trip.   1   2   3   4   5

19. I recognize new strengths I possess because of the experiential trip.   1   2   3   4   5

20. I use the challenge by choice philosophy in my life post trip.   1   2   3   4   5

21. I would recommend this experience to someone with similar life experiences as me.   1   2   3   4   5

22. I would recommend this experience to a friend/family member.   1   2   3   4   5

23. What was the most impactful part of your experience?

24. What was the least helpful part of your experience?

25. How did the wilderness/nature influence your healing on this trip?

26. Other comments???

Conclusions

We hope that you can integrate the theory, principles, and skills of Experiential Therapy into your own practice. We have truly enjoyed sharing with you our life work and passion. We would like to extend an invitation from us to customize a training or in-service on Experiential Therapy at your organization or for a consultation to begin or to fine-tune your Experiential Therapy practice. Our email is ExperientialTherapyForALL@gmail.com.

We hope to see you outdoors!

References

Alkema, K., Linton, J. M., & Davies, R. (2008). A study of the relationship between self-care, compassion satisfaction, compassion fatigue, and burnout among hospice professionals. Journal of Social Work in End-of-Life & Palliative Care, 4(2), 101–119.

American Psychiatric Association. (2013). Diagnostic and statistical manual of mental disorders (5th ed.; DSM-5). Arlington, VA: Author.

Atchley, R. A., Strayer, D. L., & Atchley, P. (2012). Creativity in the wild: Improving creative reasoning through immersion in natural settings. PLoS ONE, 7(12), e51474. doi:10.1371/journal.pone.0051474.

Attachment & Trauma Network (ATN). (2024). Trauma-aware: Definition. https://www.attachmenttraumanetwork.org/trauma-aware-definition/.

Barnes, J. E., Noll, J. G., Putnam, F. W., & Trickett, P. K. (2009). Sexual and physical revictimization among victims of severe childhood sexual abuse. Child Abuse and Neglect, 33, 412–420.

Barrows, A. (1995). The ecopsychology of child development. In T. Roszak, M. Gomes, & A. Kanner (Eds.), Ecopsychology (pp. 101–110). San Francisco, CA: Sierra Club Books.

Bartlett, J. (2021). Trauma-informed practices in early childhood education. ZERO TO THREE, 41(3), 24–34.

Barton, J., & Pretty, J. (2010). What is the best dose of nature and green exercise for improving mental health? A multi-study analysis. Environ Sci Technol, 44(10), 3947–3955. doi: 10.1021/es903183r.PMID:20337470.

Beauchemin, J., Hutchins, T. L., Patterson, F. (2008). Mindfulness Meditation May Lessen Anxiety, Promote Social Skills, and Improve Academic Performance Among Adolescents with Learning Disabilities. Complementary health practice review, 13(1), 34–45. doi:10.1177/1533210107311624.

Beck, D. (2016). Mindfulness: 10 lessons in self-care for social workers. The New Social Worker. http://www.socialworker.com/feature-articles/practice/mindfulness-10-lessons-in-self-care-for-social-workers/.

Beck, D. (2020). Re-examining mindfulness: A tool for self-care during the coronavirus crisis and beyond. The New Social Worker. https://www.socialworker.com/feature-articles/practice/reexamining-mindfulness-tool-self-care-during-coronavirus-crisis-beyond. https://doi.org/10.1080/15524250802353934.

Bloomquist, K., Wood, L., Freidmeyer-Trainer, K., & Kim, H. (2015). Self-care and professional quality of life: Predictive factors among MSW practitioners. Advances in Social Work, 16(2), 292–311. doi:10.18060/18760.

Borton, T. (1970). Reach, touch and teach. New York: McGraw-Hill Paperbacks.

Bratman, G., Hamilton, P., Hahn, K., Daily, G., & Gross, J. (2015). Nature experience reduces rumination and subgenual prefrontal cortex activation. PNAS, 112(28), 8567–8572. www.pnas.org/cgi/doi/10.1073/pnas.1510459112.

Briere, J. (2002). Treating adult survivors of severe childhood abuse and neglect: Further development of an integrative model. In J. E. B. Myers, L. Berliner, J. Briere, C. T. Hendrix, T. Reid, & C. Jenny (Eds.), The APSAC handbook on child maltreatment (2nd ed., pp. 175–204). Newbury Park, CA: Sage Publications.

Bronfenbrenner, U. (1979). The ecology of human development. Cambridge, MA: Harvard University Press.

Bronfenbrenner, U. (1986). Ecology of the family as a context for human development: Research perspectives. Developmental Psychology, 22(6), 723–742.

Bronfenbrenner, U. (1989). Ecological systems theory. Annals of Child Development, 6, 723–742.

Bubolz, M., & Sontag, S. (1993). Human ecology theory. In P. Boss, W. Doherty, R. LaRossa, W. Schumm, & S. Steinmetz (Eds.), Sourcebook of family theories and methods: A contextual approach (pp. 419–448). New York: Plenum Press.

Buzzell, L., & Chalquist, C. (2009). Ecotherapy. Berkeley, CA: Counterpoint.

Caron, C. (2024, February 5). Therapists trade the couch for the great outdoors. New York Times. https://www.nytimes.com/2024/02/05/well/mind/outdoors-therapy-depression-anxiety.html.

Cassella, C. (2020). Daycares in Finland built a "forest floor," and it changed children's immune systems. Science Advances. https://www.sciencealert.com/daycares-in-finlandbuiltabacky ar...id=IwAR1cjV4z4V_OJgPpOpRzQdlumenBAeg8xr5eKx8le5IFGeKcNzHoVZtA8.

Centers for Disease Control and Prevention (CDC). (n.d.). Fast facts: Preventing adverse childhood experiences. https://www.cdc.gov/violenceprevention/aces/fastfact.html.

Christiana, R., Battista, R., James, J., & Bergman, S. (2017). Pediatrician prescriptions for outdoor physical activity among children: A pilot study. Preventive Medicine, 5, 100–105. doi: 10.1016/j.pmedr.2016.12.005.https://www.ncbi.nlm.nih.gov/pmc/articles/PMC5153440/.

Chun, M. H., Chang, M. C., & Lee, S. (2017). The effects of forest therapy on depression and anxiety in patients with chronic stroke. International Journal of Neuroscience, 127(3), 199–203. doi.org/10.3109/00207454.2016.1170015.

Colzato, L. S., Ozturk, A., & Hommel, B. (2012). Meditate to create: The impact of focused-attention and open-monitoring training on convergent and divergent thinking. Frontiers in Psychology, 3, 116. https://doi.org/10.3389/fpsyg.2012.00116.

Connolly, K., & Sullivan, M. (n.d.). Community resilience model: Introduction. Trauma Resource Institute. Health Federation of Philadelphia. https://forbetterhealthpa.org/wp-content/uploads/2018/05/PBH-5-1-18-CRM-Slides-1.pdf.

Cronin, C., Forsstrom, M., & Papageorge, N. (2020). What good are treatment effects without treatment? Mental health and the reluctance to use talk therapy. National Bureau of Economic Research, 27711. doi:10.3386/w27711. https://www.nber.org/papers/w27711.

Dahl, C. J., Wilson-Mendenhall, C. D., & Davidson, R. J. (2020). The plasticity of well-being: A training-based framework for the cultivation of human flourishing. Proceedings of the National Academy of Sciences, 117(51), 32197–32206. https://doi.org/10.1073/pnas. 2014859117.

Dalphon, H. (2019). Self-care techniques for social workers: Achieving an ethical harmony between work and well-being. Journal of Human Behavior in the Social Environment, 29(1), 85–95. https://doi.10.1080/10911359.2018.1481802.

Desbordes, G., Lobsang T., Thaddeus, N., Pace, B. Wallace, A., Raison, C., & Schwartz E. (2012). Effects of mindful-attention and compassion meditation training on amygdala response to emotional stimuli in an ordinary, non-meditative state. Frontiers in Human Neuroscience, 6, 292–307. doi:10.3389/fnhum.2012.00292.

Dewey, J. (1939). Experience and education: The Kappa Delta Pi lecture series. New York: Collier Books Macmillan.

Duncan, B., Miller, S., Wampold, B. & Hubble, M. (2010). The heart and soul of change, 2nd edition: Delivering what works in therapy. Washington, DC: American Psychological Association.

Dweck, C. (2007). Mindset: The new psychology of success. New York: Ballantine Books.

Eastwood, C. D., & Ecklund, K., (2008). Compassion fatigue risk and self-care practices among residential treatment center childcare workers. Residential Treatment For Children & Youth, *25*(2), 103–122. doi: 10.1080/08865710802309972.

Edwards, M., Adams, E. M., Waldo, M., Hadfield, O. D., & Biegel, G. M. (2014). Effects of a mindfulness group on Latino adolescent students: Examining levels of perceived stress, mindfulness, self-compassion, and psychological symptoms. The Journal for Specialists in Group Work, *39*(2), 145–163. https://doi.org/10.1080/01933922.2014.891683.

Emerson, D., & Hopper, E. (2011). Overcoming trauma through yoga: Reclaiming your body. Berkeley, CA: North Atlantic Books.

Feldscher, K. (2018, November 6). Training your mind to improve well-being. *Harvard T.H. Chan School of Public Health.* https://www.hsph.harvard.edu/news/features/richard-davidson-well-being/#:~:text=Davidson%20outlined%20four%20components%20of, promoting%20changes%20inside%20the%20brain.

Feng, X., Mosimah, C., Sizemore, G., Goyat, R. & Dwibedi, N. (2019). Impact of mindful self-care and perceived stress on the health related quality of life among young-adult students in West Virginia. *Journal of Human Behavior in the Social Environment, 29*(1), 26–36. doi:10.1080/10911359.2018.1470953.

Finkelhor, D., Ormrod, R., & Turner, H. (2009). Lifetime assessment of poly-victimization in a national sample of children and youth. Child Abuse and Neglect, *33*(7), 403–411.

Finkelhor, D., Ormrod, R. K., & Turner, H. A. (2007). Polyvictimization and trauma in a national longitudinal cohort. Development and psychopathology, *19*(1), 149–166. https://doi.org/10.1017/S0954579407070083.

Finkelhor, D., Ormrod, R., Turner, H., & Hamby, S. L. (2005). The victimization of children and youth: A comprehensive, national survey. Child Maltreatment, *10*(1), 5–25.

Fisher, C. (2023). Trauma-informed nature therapy: A case study. Ecopsychology, *15*(3), 214–221.

Flom, J. A. (2022). Toward an anti-oppressive, trauma-informed, practice in outdoor therapies. Master's thesis, University of the Fraser Valley.

Ford, J., & Hawke, J. (2012). Trauma affect regulation psychoeducation group attendance is associated with reduced disciplinary incidents and sanctions in juvenile detention facilities. Journal of Aggression, Maltreatment, and Trauma, *21*, 365–384. https://doi.org/fmn5.

Freedenthal, S. (2021). Suicidal thoughts and related behavior. In J. Laser & N. Nicotera (Eds.), Working with adolescents: A clinical guide for practitioners (2nd ed., pp. 253–269). New York: Guilford Press.

Furuyashiki, A., Tabuchi, K., Norikoshi, K., Kobayashi, T., & Oriyama, S. (2019). A comparative study of the physiological and psychological effects of forest bathing (Shinrin-yoku) on working age people with and without depressive tendencies. Environmental Health and Preventative Medicine, *24*(1), 46–57. doi:10.1186/s12199-019-0800-1.

Germer, C., & Neff, K. (2019). Teaching the mindful self-compassion program: A guide for professionals. New York: Guilford Press.

Goldsmith, H. (1998). The way: An ecological world view. Athens: University of Georgia Press.

Grasse, J. (2023). Healing hikes of Door County. Sister Bay, WI: Innovative Printing.

Great Pedagogical Thinkers. (2023). https://www.pedagogy4change.org/john-dewey//

Greenland, S. (2012). *Teaching the ABC's of attention, balance, and compassion.* TEDx Talks: TEDxStudioCityED. https://www.youtube.com/watch?v=LpMvTTIr2p4

Greeson, J., Juberg, M., Maytan, M., James, K. & Rogers, H. (2014). A randomized controlled trial of Koru: A mindfulness program for college students and other emerging adults. Journal of American College Health, *62*(4), 222–233. doi:10.1080/07448481.2014.887571.

Griffore, R. & Phenice, L. (2001). The language of human ecology. Dubuque, IA: Kendall/Hunt.

Grise-Owens, G., Miller, J., & Eaves, M. (Eds.). (2016). The A-to-Z self-care handbook for social workers and other helping professionals. The New Social Worker Press.

Han, J., Choi, H., Jeon, Y., Yoon, C., Woo, J., Kim, W. (2016). The effects of forest therapy on coping with chronic widespread pain: Physiological and psychological differences between participants in a forest therapy program and a control group. International Journal of Environmental Research and Public Health, 13(3), 255–268. doi:10.3390/ijerph13030255.

Hanh, T. (1997). Interview with Terry Gross. Fresh Air, National Public Radio. https://www.freshair.com/segments/writer-and-peace-activist-thich-nhat-hanh.

Hanh, T. (2015). Silence: The power of quiet in a world full of noise. New York: Harper One.

Hanscom, A. (2016). Balanced and barefoot: How unrestricted outdoor play makes for strong, confident capable children. Oakland, CA: New Harbinger Publications.

Harker, R. Pidgeon, A., Klaassen, F. and King, S. (2016). Exploring resilience and mindfulness as preventative factors for psychological distress burnout and secondary traumatic stress among human service professionals. Work, 54(3), 631–637. https://doi:10.3233/WOR-162311.

Harper, N. (2017). Wilderness therapy, therapeutic camping and adventure education in child and youth care literature: A scoping review. Children and Youth Services Review 83, 68–79. doi:10.1016/j.childyouth.2017.10.030.

Harper, N. J., Fernee, C. R., & Gabrielsen, L. E. (2021). Nature's role in outdoor therapies: An umbrella review. International Journal of Environmental Research and Public Health, 18, 5117. https://doi.org/10.3390/ijerph18105117.

Hayword, T. (1994). Ecological thought. Cambridge, UK: Polity Press.

Healthy Minds Innovations. (n.d.). Sound cloud recording Open Awareness 5-minute seated meditation. https://soundcloud.com/user-984650879/open-awareness-cort-5-min-seated.

Herman, J. (1992). Trauma and recovery. New York: Basic Books.

Herman, J. (2015). Trauma and recovery (rev. ed.). New York: Basic Books.

Hershler, A. (2021). Window of tolerance. In Hershler, A., Hughes, L., Nguyen, P., & Wall, S. (Eds.), Looking at trauma: A tool kit for clinicians (Vol. 23; pp. 25–28). University Park: Penn State University Press. https://doi.org/10.5325/j.ctv1wmz3qr.

Hill, C. E., & Norcross, J. C. (Eds.). (2023). Psychotherapy skills and methods that work. New York: Oxford University Press.

Howell, A. & Buro, K. (2011). Relations Among Mindfulness, Achievement-Related Self-Regulation, and Achievement Emotions. Journal of Happiness Studies, 12(6), 1007–1022. DOI: 10.1007/s10902-010-9241-7.

Ideno, Y., Hayashi, K., Abe, Y., Ueda, K., Iso, H., Noda, M., Lee, J. & Suzuk, S. (2017). Blood pressure-lowering effect of Shinrin-yoku (Forest bathing): A systematic review and meta-analysis. BMC Complementary and Alternative Medicine, 17, 409–421. doi.org/10.1186/s12906-017-1912-z.

Improvised Life (n.d.). Jung, C. Dream analysis: Notes on a lecture given in 1928–193). https://improvisedlife.com/2020/08/17/carl-jung-and-mary-oliver-on-touching-nature-from-the-inside-and-outside/.

Jha, A. (2018). How to tame your wandering mind. Ted Talk. https://www.ted.com/talks/amishi_jha_how_to_tame_your_wandering_mind?subtitle=en

Johnson, E. G., Davis, E. B., Johnson, J., Pressley, J. D., Sawyer, S., & Spinazzola, J. (2020). The effectiveness of trauma-informed wilderness therapy with adolescents: A pilot study. Psychological Trauma: Theory, Research, Practice, and Policy, 12(8), 878–887. https://doi.org/10.1037/tra0000595.

Jones, K. (2023, March 20). The multitasking myth. Evidence Based Education. https://evidencebased.education/the-multitasking-myth/#:~:text=Multitasking%20is%20a%20myth%20because,from%20one%20task%20to%20another.

Jorgensen, A. (2020, August 6). What are green prescriptions and how do they work? *World Economic Forum*. https://www.weforum.org/agenda/2020/08/green-prescriptionshwAR05seMSnbvLPr0H4_7QNwWTELSH06wDWOfZGpt3kKoHg6cHYav3kXk_00.

Joschko, L., Pálsdóttir, A., Grahn P., & Hinse, M. (2023). Nature-based therapy in individuals with mental health disorders, with a focus on mental well-being and connectedness to nature: A pilot study. International Journal of Environmental Research and Public Health, *20*, 2167–2191. https://doi.org/10.3390/ijerph20032167.

Kabat-Zinn, J. (2013). Full catastrophe living (revised edition): Using the wisdom of your body and mind to face stress, pain, and illness. New York: Bantam Books.

Kabat-Zinn, J. (2021). Meditation is not what you think. Mindfulness, *12*(3), 784–787. https://doi.org/10.1007/s12671-020-01578-1.

Kaplan. A. (2020, January 29). Does science support the "wilderness" in wilderness therapy? *Undark*. https://undark.org/2020/01/29/does-science-support-the-wildern...ctzQeUxLcRRa4FZJmTlUc554LKpEwidXqVU3VpuwKK9q7E&_hsmi=82710885.

Keltner, D. (2024). Awe, the new science of everyday wonder and how it can transform your life. New York: Penguin Books.

Kessler, D. (2020). Finding meaning: The sixth stage of grief. New York: Scribner Books.

Kessler, D. (2023, Spring). Grief Educator Training. https://grief.com.

Kettler, A. (April 8, 2016). Doctors explain how hiking actually changes our brains. *Collective Evolution*. https://www.collective-evolution.com/2016/04/08/doctorsexplain...=IwAR18oUTnebZosMaNMXtSWKU6MT5Qw138TiDGu4fz4lxF19FIzfTMut.

Kilpatrick, D., Resnick, H., Milanak, M., Miller, M., Keyes, K. & Friedman, M. (2013). National estimates of exposure to traumatic events and PTSD prevalence using DSM-IV and DSM-5 criteria. Journal of Traumatic Stress, *26*(5), 537–547.

Klimes, W. & Klimes, M. (1986). *John Muir: A Reading Bibliography by Kimes, 1986 (Muir articles 1866–1986)*. Panorama West Books.

Knutson, T. (2023). https://www.traceyknutson.com.

Kraemer, K., Luberto, C., O'Bryan, E., Mysinger, E., & Cotton, S. (2016). Mind–body skills training to improve distress tolerance in medical students: A pilot study. Teaching and Learning in Medicine, *28*(2), 219–228. doi:10.1080/10401334.2016.1146605.

Kral, T., Schuyler, B., Mumford, J., Rosenkranz, M., Lutza, A., & Davidson, R. (2018). Impact of short- and long-term mindfulness meditation training on amygdala reactivity to emotional stimuli. Neuroimage, *181*, 301–313. doi:10.1016/j.neuroimage.2018.07.013.

Kuo, F. & Taylor, A. (2004). A potential natural treatment for attention-deficit/hyperactivity disorder: Evidence from a national study. American Journal of Public Health, *94*(9), 1580–1586.

Kyeong, L. (2013). Self-compassion as a moderator of the relationship between academic burn- out and psychological health in Korean cyber university students. Personality and Individual Differences, *54*, 899–902. doi:10.1016/J.PAID.2013.01.001.

Lahav, Y., & Elklit, A. (2016). The cycle of healing: Dissociation and attachment during treatment of CSA survivors. Child Abuse and Neglect, *60*, 67–76.

Landres, P., Vagias, W., & Stutzman, S. (2012). Using wilderness character to improve wilderness stewardship. Park Science, *28*, 3. https://research.fs.usda.gov/treesearch/40396.

Laser, J. (2022). Evaluating the individual and group outcomes of individuals who participated in experiential therapy activities at a challenge course. International Journal of Social Work, *9*, 26–33. doi:10.5296/ijsw.v9i1.19308.

Laser, J., & Nicotera, N. (2021). Working with adolescents: A clinical guide for practitioners (2nd ed.). New York: Guilford Press.

Laser, J., Petersen, G., Stephens, H., DeRito, D., & Boeckel, J. (2019). Demographics, risk factors, and negative historical events of inpatients with a history of sexual abuse. Advances in Social Sciences Research Journal (ASSRJ), 6(10), 184–194. doi:10.14738/assrj. 610.7269.

Laser, J., & Stephens, P. (2011). Working with military families through deployment and beyond. Clinical Social Work Journal, 39(1), 28–38. doi:10.1007/s10615-010-0310-5.

Laser, J., & Wallis, D. (2014). Outpatient family systems therapy as the treatment modality for adolescent substance abuse. Addiction, Recovery and Aftercare, 1(1), 69–84.

Laser-Maira, J. (2016). Children's experiential therapy group in an elementary school. In W. Pelech, R. Basso, C. Lee, & M. Gandarilla (Eds.), Inclusive group work (pp. 231–246). New York: Oxford University Press.

Laser-Maira, J., Blair, D., Blair Echevarria, J., Wallis, D., Castro, O., & Conger, J. (2019). Youth and their families: A guide to treating adolescent substance use through family systems therapy. New York: Oxford University Press.

Laser-Maira, J. A., Hounmenou, C., & Peach, D. (2020). Global commercial and sexual exploitation of children. In E. Erez & P. Ibarra (Eds.), Oxford Encyclopedia of International Criminology (pp. 43–63). New York and Oxford: Oxford University Press. https://doi.org/ 10.1093/acrefore/9780190264079.013.592.

Laser-Maira, J., Huey, C., Castro, O., & Ehrlich, K. (2016). Human trafficking in Peru: Stakeholder perceptions. International Social Work Journal, 3(1), 50–64. http://dx.doi.org/10. 5296/ijsw.v3i1.8750.

Laser-Maira, J., Huey, C., Castro, O., Ehrlich, K., & Nicotera, N. (2018). Human trafficking in Peru: Stakeholder perceptions of how to combat human trafficking and help support its survivors. Journal of Sociology and Social Work, 6(1), 34–40. ISSN: 2333-5807 (Print), 2333-5815 (Online).

Laser-Maira, J., & Nicotera, N. (2019). Innovative skills to increase cohesion and communication in couples. New York: Oxford University Press.

Laser-Maira, J, Peach, D., & Hounmenou, C. (2019). Moving towards self-actualization: A trauma-informed and needs-focused approach to the mental health needs of survivors of commercial child sexual exploitation. International Journal of Social Work, 6(2), 27–34. https://doi.org/10.5296/ijsw.v6i2.15198.

Lawson, G., & Myers, J. (2011). Wellness, professional quality of life, and career-sustaining behaviors: What keeps us well? Journal of Counseling and Development, 89(2), 163–171. https://doi:10.1002/j.1556-6678.2011.tb00074.x.

Lay, K. (2016). Mindfulness. In G. Grise-Owens, J. Miller, & M. Eaves. (Eds.), The A-to-Z self-care handbook for social workers and other helping professionals (pp. 80–84). The New Social Worker Press.

Le, T. N., & Proulx, J. (2015). Feasibility of mindfulness-based intervention for incarcerated mixed-ethnic Native Hawaiian/Pacific Islander youth. Asian American Journal of Psychology, 6(2), 181. https://doi.org/10.1037/aap0000019.

Leave No Trace. (2021). Center for Outdoor Ethics. https://lnt.org/why/7-principles/.

Lee, J. (2020). What's in your backpack? Mindful self-care and emotional rigor during the COVID-19 crisis. The New Social Worker. https://www.socialworker.com/feature-articles/ practice/your-backpack-mindful-self-care-emotional-rigor-covid19-crisis/.

Lee, M. Y., Ng, S. M., Leung, P. P. Y., & Chan, C. L. W. (2009). Integrative body-mind-spirit social work: An empirically based approach to assessment and treatment. New York: Oxford University Press.

Leitch, L. (2017). Action steps using ACEs and trauma-informed care: A resilience model. Health Justice, 5, Article 5. https://doi.org/10.1186/s40352-017-0050-5.

Leitch, M., Vanslyke, J., & Allen, M. (2009). Somatic experiencing treatment with social service workers following hurricanes Katrina and Rita. Social Work, 54(1), 9–18. https://doi.org/fxwccd.

Levine, P. (1997). Waking the tiger: Healing trauma: The innate capacity to transform overwhelming experiences. North Atlantic Books.

Levine, P. (2010). In an unspoken voice: How the body releases trauma and restores goodness North Atlantic Books.

Louv, R. (2008). Last child in the woods. Chapel Hill, NC: Algonquin Books.

Lu, D., Palmer, J. R., Rosenberg, L., Shields, A. E., Orr, E. H., DeVivo, I., & Cozier, Y. C. (2019). Perceived racism in relation to telomere length among African American women in the Black Women's Health Study. Annals of Epidemiology, 36, 33–39. https://doi.org/10.1016/j.annepidem.2019.06.003.

Lutz, A., Slagter, H. A., Dunne, J. D., & Davidson, R. J. (2008). Attention regulation and monitoring in meditation. Trends in Cognitive Sciences, 12(4), 163–169. https://doi.org/10.1016/j.tics.2008.01.005.

Maddock, A., McCusker, P., Blair, C., & Roulston, A. (2021). The mindfulness-based social work and self-care programme: A mixed methods evaluation study. British Journal of Social Work, 52(5), 2760–2777. doi.org/10.1093/bjsw/bcab203.

Marchand, W. R. (2014). Neural mechanisms of mindfulness and meditation: Evidence from neuroimaging studies. World journal of radiology, 6(7), 471–479. https://doi.org/10.4329/wjr.v6.i7.471.

Mark, G., Gudith, D., & Klocke, U. (2008). The cost of interrupted work. Proceedings of the SIGCHI Conference on Human Factors in Computing Systems, 107–110. https://doi.org/10.1145/1357054.1357072.

Mathews. F. (1991). The ecological self. Savage, MD: Barnes and Noble Books.

McConnico, N., Boynton-Jarrett, R., Bailey, C., & Nandi, M. (2016). A framework for trauma sensitive schools: Infusing trauma-informed practices into early childhood education systems. ZERO TO THREE, 36(5), 36–44. https://www.zerotothree.org/resources/series/journal-archive.

Menakem, R. (2017). My grandmother's hands: Racialized trauma and the pathway to mending our hearts and bodies. Las Vagas, NV: Central Recovery Press.

Mendelson, T., Greenberg, M., Dariotis, J., Feagans Gould, L., Rhoades, B., & Leaf, P. (2010). Feasibility and preliminary outcomes of a school-based mindfulness intervention for urban youth. Journal of Abnormal Child Psychology, 38, 985–994. doi:10.1007/s10802-010-9418-x.

Merchant, C. (1999). Ecology: Key concepts and critical theory. Amherst, NY: Humanity Books.

Meredith, G. R., Rakow, D. A., Eldermire, E. R., Madsen, C. G., Shelley, S. P., & Sachs, N. A. (2020). Minimum time dose in nature to positively impact the mental health of college-aged students, and how to measure it: A scoping review. Frontiers in psychology, 10, 2942. https://doi.org/10.3389/fpsyg.2019.02942.

Mina, A. (2023, February 5). The Buddhist monk who brought mindfulness to the West. https://hyperallergic.com/798230/buddhist-monk-thich-nhat-hanh-who-brought-mindfulness-to-the-west/.

Mindremapping Academy. (2023). Difference between trauma aware, trauma sensitive, trauma informed, and trauma responsive: Understanding the nuances. https://mindremappingacademy.com/difference-between-trauma-aware-trauma-sensitive-trauma-informed-and-trauma-responsive-understanding-the-nuances-2/.

Moniuzko, S. (2022, December 8). Wilderness therapy was supposed to help these "troubled teens." It traumatized them instead. *USA Today*. https://www.usatoday.com/in-depth/life/healthwellness/2022/12/08/wilderness-therapy-troubled-teen-industry/9890694002/.

Musheer, M. (2021). The trigger scale. In Hershler, A., Hughes, L., Nguyen, P., & Wall, S. (Eds.), Looking at trauma: A tool kit for clinicians (Vol. 23, pp. 29–33). University Park: Penn State University Press. https://doi.org/10.5325/j.ctv1wmz3qr.

Najavits, L. (2002). Seeking safety: A treatment manual for PTSD and substance abuse. New York: Guilford Press.

National Institute for the Clinical Application of Behavioral Medicine. (2019). *How trauma can affect your window of tolerance*. https://nicabmstealthseminar.s3.amazonaws.com/Infographics/window-of-tolerance/NICABM-InfoG-window-of-tolerance.jpg.

Neff, K. (2003). Self-compassion: An alternative conceptualization of a healthy attitude toward oneself. *Self and Identity*, 2, 85–103. doi:10.1080/15298860390129863.

Neff, K., & Germer, C. (2013). A pilot study and randomized controlled trial of the mindful self-compassion program. Journal of Clinical Psychology, 69(1), 28–44.

Nghiem, D. (2021). Flowers in the dark: Reclaiming your power to heal from trauma with mindfulness. Berkeley, CA: Parallax Press.

Nicotera, N., & Laser, J. (2019, December 6). What is well-being? Accepting strengths and foibles. *Psychology Today*. https://www.psychologytoday.com/us/blog/innovating-resiliency/201912/what-is-well-being.

Nicotera, N., & Laser-Maira, J. (2017). Innovative skills to support well-being and resiliency in youth. New York, NY: Oxford University Press.

Norton, C., Tucker, A., Rupe, B., & Riley, M.(2023). Positive youth development and adventure therapy with underserved youth: An evaluation of the Chicago Voyagers Program. Journal of Outdoor Recreation, Education, and Leadership, 15(4), 48–65. https://doi.org/10.18666/JOREL-2023-1170.

Ogden, P., Minton, K., & Pain, C. (2006). Trauma and the body: A sensorimotor approach to psychotherapy. New York: W. W. Norton.

Okoren, N. (2022, November 14). Programs purport to teach teenagers struggling with mental health problems to learn choice and accountability through powers of nature, with little oversight. *The Guardian*. https://www.theguardian.com/us-news/2022/nov/14/uswilderness-therapy-camps-troubled-teen-industry-abuse.

Ozawa-de Silva, B. (2023, November 14). Embodied healing lessons on how to listen to the body, create safe spaces, and learn new ways of being. *Insights: Journey into the heart of contemplative science*. Mind and Life Institute. https://www.mindandlife.org/insight/embodied-healing/.

Plotkin, B. (2013). Wild mind: A field guide to the human psyche. New World Library.

Pollack, S., Pedulla, T. & Siegel, R. (2014). Sitting together: Essential skills for mindfulness-based psychotherapy. New York: Guilford Press.

Prochaska, J. O., DiClemente, C. C., & Norcross, J. C. (1992). In search of how people change: Applications to addictive behaviors. American Psychologist, 47, 1102–1114.

Radey, M., & Figley, C. (2007). The social psychology of compassion. Clinical Social Work Journal, 35, 207–214. https://doi.org/10.1007/s10615-007-0087-3.

Rogers, H., & Maytan, M. (2019). Mindfulness for the next generation: Helping emerging adults manage stress and lead healthier lives (2nd ed.). New York: Oxford University Press.

Rohnke, K. (1977). Cowstails and cobras. Hamilton, MA: Project Adventure.

Rohnke, K. (1984). Silver bullets. Hamilton, MA: Project Adventure.

Rose, K. (2024). Colorado Ecotherapy Institute. http://www.coloradoecotherapyinstitute.com.

Rose, L., Williams, I., Ollson, C., & Allen, N. (2018). Promoting adolescent health and well being through outdoor youth programs: Results from a multisite Australian study. Journal of Outdoor Recreation, Education, and Leadership, *10*(1), 33–51. https://doi.org/10.18666/JOREL-2018-V10-I1-8087.

Roszak, T., Gomes, M., & Kanner, A. (1995). Ecopsychology. San Francisco, CA: Sierra Club Books.

Rothschild, B. (2011). Trauma essentials: The go-to guide. New York: W. W. Norton.

Sakre, N. (2021, November 2). The hidden abuse of teen wilderness therapy. *Achona.* https://achonaonline.com/features/2021/11/the-hidden-abuse-of-teen-wilderness-therapy/.

Salmon, P. (2020). Mindful Movement in Psychotherapy. Guildford Press.

Sawyer, P., Major, B., Casad, B., Townsend, S., & Mendes, W. (2012). Discrimination and the stress response: Psychological and physiological consequences of anticipating prejudice in interethnic interactions. American Journal of Public Health, *102*(5), 1020–1026.

Schell, L., Cotton, S., & Luxmoore, M. (2012). Outdoor adventure for young people with a mental illness: Outdoor adventure for young people. Early Intervention in Psychiatry, *6*(4), 407–414. https://doi.org/10.1111/j.1751-7893.2011.00326.x.

Selhub, E., & Logan, A. (2012). Your brain on nature. Toronto, CA: HarperCollins Publisher.

Sessions, G. (1995). Deep ecology for the 21st century. Boston, MA: Shambala.

Shao, R., & Skarlicki, D. (2009). The role of mindfulness in predicting individual performance. Canadian Journal of Behavioural Science, *41*(4), 195–201. doi:10.1037/a0015166.

Sheets, R. (2022, January 4). America's controversial "troubled teen" wilderness therapy camps—and why survivors like Paris Hilton want to stop them. *The Independent.* https://www.independent.co.uk/news/world/americas/wilderness-therapy-camps-parishilton-b1984632.html.

Shin, L., McNally, R., Kosslyn, S., Thompson, W., Rauch, S., Alpert, N., Metzger, R., Lasko, N., Orr, S. & Pittman, R. (1999). Regional cerebral blood flow during script-driven imagery in childhood sexual abuse–related posttraumatic stress disorder: A PET investigation. American Journal of Psychiatry, *156*, 575–584.

Siegel, D. (1999). The developing mind (Vol. 296). New York: Guilford Press.

Siegel, D. (2012). The developing mind: How relationships and the brain interact to shape who we are (2nd ed.). New York: Guilford Press.

Stamm, B. (2009–2012). *Professional quality of life: Compassion satisfaction and fatigue, Version 5 (ProQOL).* www.proqol.org.

Stamm, B. (2010). *The concise manual for the professional quality of life scale.* https://web.archive.org/web/20180721220000id_/https://nbpsa.org/images/PRP/ProQOL_Concise_2ndEd_12-2010.pdf.

Sternberg, R. J. (1986). A triangular theory of love. Psychological Review, *93*, 119–135.

Stillman, J. (2020, January 30). Neuroscientist: To keep your brain young, go hiking. *Inc.com.* https://www.inc.com/jessica-stillman/neuroscientist-to-keepyou...d=IwAR3QT6lP4eoE9OPrxgDT567lLkEHSMqxl7t8J2HST4U6CQ4sMLDmIVXNog.

Stoller, C. C., Greuel, J. H., Cimini, L. S., Fowler, M. S., & Koomar, J. A. (2012). Effects of sensory-enhanced yoga on symptoms of combat stress in deployed military personnel. The American Journal of Occupational Therapy, *66*(1), 59–68.

Substance Abuse and Mental Health Services Administration. (2014). SAMHSA's concept of trauma and guidance for a trauma-informed approach. HHS Publication No. (SMA) 14-4884. Rockville, MD: Author.

Substance Abuse and Mental Health Services Administration (SAMHSA). (2019). Mental health and substance use disorders. Retrieved from www.samhsa.gov/find-help/disorders.

Sue, D. (2010). Microaggressions in everyday life: Race, gender, sexual orientation. New York; John Wiley & Sons.

Sue, D. W., Alsaidi, S., Awad, M. N., Glaeser, E., Calle, C. Z., & Mendez, N. (2019). Disarming racial microaggressions: Microintervention strategies for targets, White allies, and bystanders. American Psychologist, 74(1), 128–142. https://doi.org/10.1037/amp0000296.

Swedo, E., Aslam, M., Dahlberg, L., Niolon, P., Guinn, A., Simon, T. & Mercy, J. (2023). Prevalence of adverse childhood experiences among U.S. adults: Behavioral risk factor surveillance system, 2011–2020. Morbidity Mortality Weekly Report (MMWR), 72, 707–715. http://dx.doi.org/10.15585/mmwr.mm7226a2.

Tambyah, R., Olcoń, K., Allan, J., Destry, P., & Astell-Burt, T. (2022). Mental health clinicians' perceptions of nature-based interventions within community mental health services: Evidence from Australia. BMC Health Services Research, 22, 841. https://doi.org/10.1186/s12913-022-08223-8.

The Tapping Solution Foundation. (2024). https://www.tappingsolutionfoundation.org/howdoesitwork/.

Tatum, B. (1997). Why are all the Black kids sitting together in the cafeteria? And other conversations about race. New York: Basic Books.

Thieleman, K., & Cacciatore, J. (2014). Witness to suffering: Mindfulness and compassion fatigue among traumatic bereavement volunteers and professionals. Social Work, 59, 34–41. doi:10.1093/sw/swt044.

Thomas, J., & Otis, M. (2010). Intrapsychic correlates of professional quality of life: Mindfulness, empathy, and emotional separation. Journal of the Society for Social Work and Research, 1, 83–98. doi:10.5243/jsswr.2010.7.

Thomas, J. (2012). Does personal distress mediate the effect of mindfulness on professional quality of life? Advances in Social Work, 13(3), 561–585. doi:10.18060/2600.

Thomashow, M. (1995). Ecological identity: becoming a reflective environmentalist. Boston, MA: Massachusetts Institute of Technology Press.

Thompson, I., Amatea, E., & Thompson, E. (2014). Personal and contextual predictors of mental health counselors' compassion fatigue and burnout. Journal of Mental Health Counseling, 36, 58–77. doi:10.17744/mehc.36.1.p61m73373m4617r3.

Toomey, R. B., & Anhalt, K. (2016). Mindfulness as a coping strategy for bias-based school victimization among Latina/o sexual minority youth. Psychology of Sexual Orientation and Gender Diversity, 3(4), 432. https://doi.org/10.1037/sgd0000192.

Treleaven, D. (2018). Trauma sensitive mindfulness: Practices for safe and transformative healing. New York: W.W. Norton.

Tsunetsugu, Y., Park, B. I., & Miyazaki, Y. (2010). Trends in research related to "Shinrinyoku" (taking in the forest atmosphere or forest bathing) in Japan. Environmental Health and Preventative Medicine, 15(1), 27–37. doi.org/10.1007/s12199-009-0091-z.

Tuckman, B. W., & Jensen, M. A. C. (1977). Stages of small-group development revisited. Group & Organization Studies, 2(4), 419–427. https://doi.org/10.1177/105960117700200404.

Uhernik, J. (2017). Using neuroscience in trauma therapy. New York: Routledge.

Van Der Kolk, B. (2014). The body keeps the score. New York: Penguin Books.

Van der Kolk, B., Stone, L., West, J., Rhodes, A., Emerson, D., Suvak, M., & Spinazzola, J. (2014). Yoga as an adjunctive treatment for posttraumatic stress disorder: A randomized controlled trial. Journal of Clinical Psychiatry, 75(6), e559–e565. https://doi.org/f59qnn.

Vygotsky, L. (1980). The mind in society: The development of higher psychological processes. Cambridge, MA: Harvard University Press.

Waelde, L. (2022). Mindfulness and meditation in trauma treatment: The inner resources for stress program. New York: Guilford Press.

Warner, E., Spinazzola. J., Westcott, A., Gunn, C., & Hodgdon, H. (2014). The body can change the score: Empirical support for somatic regulation in the treatment of traumatized adolescents. Journal Child Adolescent Trauma, 7(4), 237–246. https://doi.org/dz4t.

Warren, S., & Deckert, J. (2020). Contemplative practices for self-care in the social work classroom. Social Work, 65(1), 11–20. https://doi:10.1093/sw/swz039.

Watson, C. (2022, April 23). Massive study finds we need better therapies than antidepressants. Here's why. Science Alert. https://www.sciencealert.com/antidepressants-don-t-improve-quality-of-life-massivestudy-finds.

Wen, Y., Yan, Q., Pan, Y., Xinren Gu, & Liu, Y. (2019). Medical empirical research on forest bathing (Shinrin-yoku): A systematic review. Environmental Health and Preventative Medicine, 24, 70–91. doi.org/10.1186/s12199-019-0822-8.

Wiest, B. (n.d.). True self-care is not salt baths. Reddit. https://www.reddit.com/r/quotes/comments/10o2cbn/true_selfcare_is_not_bath_salts_and_chocolate/.

Williams, F. (2017). The nature fix: Why nature makes us happier, healthier and more creative. New York: W. W. Norton.

Wilson, L., & Wilson, H. (2004). Play to win: Choosing growth over fear in work and life. Portland, OR: Bard Press.

Women Wonder Writers. (n.d.). The balancing act: Self-care vs community care. The Write of Your Life. https://thewriteofyourlife.org/self-care-vs-community-care/?utm_term=self%20care&utm_campaig=TWOYL+-+Blog&utm_source=adwords&utm_medium=ppc&hsa_acc=3141980739&hsa_cam=10397995848&hsa_grp=121188389487&hsa_ad=497287355017&hsa_src=g&hsa_tgt=kwd-296977359344&hsa_kw=self%20care&hsa_mt=p&hsa_net=adwords&hsa_ver=3&gclid=EAIaIQobChMI5Ynpipvk9QIVdzytBh3yKAvcEAMYAiAAEgKup_D_BwE.

Yoshida, K., Takeda, K., Kasai, T., Makinae, S., Murakami, Y., Hasegawa, A., & Sakai, S. (2020). Focused attention meditation training modifies neural activity and attention: Longitudinal EEG data in non-meditators. Social Cognitive and Affective Neuroscience, 15(2), 215–224. https://doi.org/10.1093/scan/nsaa020.

Index